The
Infertility
Survival Guide

Judith C. Daniluk, Ph.D.

Foreword by Margo Fluker, M.D.

New Harbinger Publications, Inc.

Publisher's Note

Care has been taken to confirm the accuracy of the information presented and to describe generally accepted practices. However, the authors, editors, and publisher are not responsible for errors or omissions or for any consequences from application of the information in this book and make no warranty, express or implied, with respect to the contents of the publication.

The authors, editors, and publisher have exerted every effort to ensure that any drug selection and dosage set forth in this text are in accordance with current recommendations and practice at the time of publication. However, in view of ongoing research, changes in government regulations, and the constant flow of information relating to drug therapy and drug reactions, the reader is urged to check the package insert for each drug for any change in indications and dosage and for added warnings and precautions. This is particularly important when the recommended agent is a new or infrequently employed drug.

Some drugs and medical devices presented in this publication may have Food and Drug Administration (FDA) clearance for limited use in restricted research settings. It is the resposibility of the health care provider to ascertain the FDA status of each drug or device planned for use in their clinical practice.

Distributed in the U.S.A. by Publishers Group West; in Canada by Raincoast Books; in Great Britain by Airlift Book Company, Ltd.; in South Africa by Real Books, Ltd.; in Australia by Boobook; and in New Zealand by Tandem Press.

Copyright © 2001 by   Judith Daniluk
                      New Harbinger Publications, Inc.
                      5674 Shattuck Avenue
                      Oakland, CA 94609

Cover design by Lightbourne Images
Edited by Karen O'Donnell Stein
Text design by Spencer Smith

ISBN 1-57224-247-7 Paperback

Printed in the United States of America

New Harbinger Publications' Web site address: www.newharbinger.com

03   02   01

10   9   8   7   6   5   4   3   2   1

First printing

This book is dedicated to the many women and men who have taught me about the power of courage, perseverance, and hope as they faced the challenges of infertility. It has been a privilege to share your journeys.

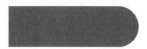

Contents

Foreword

Let's face it . . . infertility is not fun, and neither is its treatment. Nor is infertility fair. No one deserves it. Infertility does not discriminate—it affects individuals in all walks of life, regardless of age, race, culture, educational level, or income. It affects those who previously have conceived easily and it even affects infertility specialists themselves. Ironically, it seems only to spare politicians and those who make decisions about funding and access to medical treatment.

The unfulfilled desire to have a child is often the first major crisis that a couple faces in their relationship. The experience can be daunting. It has the power to erode self-esteem and destroy relationships. *But it doesn't have to be that way.* Judith Daniluk is a counseling psychologist with decades of experience helping infertile individuals and couples understand and cope. This book is filled with the wisdom she has accumulated from years of training, research, and, most importantly, from listening to women and men who are struggling with infertility.

If you are struggling with infertility, you know that you did not choose to be in this situation. *But you can choose what to do about it.* You may not be able to control the *outcome*, but you can have control over the *process*. You can become informed by seeking information from reputable sources. You can contact your local or national infertility support groups for references or direction. You can ask for advice from health care providers whom you trust and feel comfortable with. You can consider your options and make the decisions that are appropriate for your individual needs and circumstances. You can try to be prepared medically, physically, financially, and emotionally for what may lie ahead.

So how does anyone ever learn to cope? This book is filled with practical advice, both in Judith's text and in the quotes from women and men who have walked down this road ahead of you. Chapter 1 starts with the basic survival strategies: accepting that you can't control your fertility, developing realistic expectations, learning to be patient, learning to be assertive, becoming informed, trying not to blame anyone, and letting go of the expectation that it should all make sense. Chapter 2 briefly outlines infertility investigations and treatment. It is not intended to be an in-depth discussion of the specific medical details, but rather a description of what to expect and how you may feel during the process.

Chapter 3 walks you through the various hurdles you may encounter while making treatment decisions. Chapter 4 discusses strategies for coping with the stresses of treatment, including simple instructions for relaxation exercises, visualization techniques, and various other measures for managing anxiety. Chapter 7 is devoted to coping with infertility over time. Chapters 5 and 6 deal with relationships—those with your partner, your friends, your family and all the significant and insignificant others in your life who may want to know (or think they know) what you're going through. The last chapter deals with moving on.

Throughout these chapters you'll learn various strategies for understanding and coping. There is always an emphasis on keeping yourself strong and whole, on being informed, on having choices, and on making your relationship stronger because of this experience. The process involves support *from* your partner, support *for* your partner, and recognition that you are in this together, although you may have different needs, time frames, and coping strategies. Yet, in these chapters there is also the sobering acknowledgment that some women enter this process alone, while others end the journey alone because their relationships have not survived the process.

This book contains much wisdom—professional wisdom in Judith Daniluk's writing, and common sense suggestions and personal wisdom in the quotations that are interspersed throughout. Some of the quotes will make you angry. Others will make you weep. But they will all make you wiser. They will help you realize that you are not alone in this struggle . . . and that you have the power to emerge from this experience stronger and more knowledgeable about yourself, your health, and your relationships.

Margo R. Fluker, MD, FRCSC
Co-Director, Genesis Fertility Centre
Vancouver, British Columbia
Clinical Professor, Department of Obstetrics and Gynaecology
University of British Columbia

Introduction

In the early 1980s, as a doctoral student in Counseling Psychology and someone with an interest in sexuality and reproductive health, I began an internship at a fertility clinic. Infertility was not a high-profile issue at the time. Few books and articles were available about the emotional strains of being unable to produce a child. Fortunately, the coordinator of the fertility clinic was committed to finding someone to provide support to the many couples who were struggling to cope with the stresses of infertility and trying to make informed and satisfying decisions.

The year I spent working with couples in the clinic ignited a lifelong interest in assisting people to make informed and satisfying treatment and parenting decisions, deal with the stresses and invasiveness of medical treatment, and cope with their grief and loss if treatment failed. For seventeen years I've been providing psychological support to infertile individuals and couples, as well as doing research and writing articles about the struggles of infertility. Most of my writing has been focused on how mental health professionals can help their clients deal with this very challenging life experience. Many of the quotes you'll find throughout this book are the words of the women and men I've worked with over the years, as well as those who shared their stories and struggles with me during in-depth interviews as part of a three-year study funded by Health Canada (Daniluk, 1996). The study was aimed at learning more about how couples create satisfying lives when fertility treatments fail.

Little did I know when I began this work that infertility would also become a personal issue for me. Like so many others, I assumed that if, and when, I decided I wanted children I would just be able to throw away the birth control pills, and after a few months I'd get pregnant. In spite of my experience working with infertile couples, I still assumed that my fertility was under my control. However, I found out I was wrong, and I spent several difficult years trying to become a mother. I was lucky enough to have one child, but despite our best efforts and those of the medical practitioners with whom we worked, we were unable to have another. I recall only too well how difficult it was to finally give away my son's baby clothes and sell the crib and high chair, knowing that I'd never be able to use them again. I recall how painful it was to close that chapter of my life by asking my partner to have a vasectomy to help end the monthly torment.

Why Did I Write This Book?

During my own struggles and throughout the years I've been working with infertile couples, it has been difficult to find books that could help infertile clients cope with the unique stresses of medical treatments, the difficulties in making informed decisions about what to do and when to stop, the tremendous impact that being infertile makes on their significant relationships, and the ongoing uncertainty about whether they'll ever become parents. Certainly in the last ten years many good books have come out that have helped clients consider the implications of particular treatment options, such as donor sperm or donor eggs. And some have helped clients cope with adoption and the stresses of pregnancy and parenting after infertility. Some of the more current ones are listed in the Resources at the end of this book.

Clients wanted a book that provided concrete strategies for coping with infertility and medical treatment over time. Women wanted something that their partners could also relate to and find easy to read. They wanted and needed something to help them deal with the challenges of infertility and medical treatment, while maintaining their sanity, dignity, and important relationships. That's why I wrote this book.

Who Is This Book For?

This book may be helpful to anyone who must rely on the help of the medical profession to become pregnant. It is written from the perspective of women and men who are trying to produce a child together. If you are single, or a member of a lesbian couple, and you are trying to cope with the personal and relationship stresses of infertility, or the use of third-party reproductive options, you will also benefit from much of the information and many of the suggestions contained in this book.

How Can This Book Help You?

This book can help you understand and cope with infertility. It prepares you for the struggles commonly faced by infertile women and men and provides exercises and strategies to help you manage the challenges of making informed treatment decisions; coping with the stresses of medical intervention; responding to insensitive comments; handling family gatherings; fitting treatment into your life; communicating effectively with your partner; keeping your sex life alive; dealing with guilt if you're the one with the problem; coping with feelings of anger, loss, and grief; and deciding when it's time to give up treatment and move on. Arranged in an easy and readable format, each chapter is filled with the compassionate words and wisdom of other women and men who have experienced and survived infertility. Books and Web-site addresses are also listed in a resource section to help you find information and support on specific topics like in vitro fertilization; hormone therapies; and various third-party reproductive options.

Being unable to produce a child is one of the most difficult and challenging experiences in life. It is an experience filled with pain, loss, and disappointment. It is also an experience that can lead to tremendous growth and learning. It is my hope that the information and suggestions provided within each chapter will help you not only to survive infertility, but to be stronger as a person, and as a couple, as a consequence of your efforts.

Basic Survival Strategies

What Is Infertility?

Most people think of infertility as a medical condition—and it is. Infertility is usually defined as the inability to achieve a viable pregnancy (a pregnancy resulting in live birth) after twelve months of regular, unprotected intercourse.

There are essentially two types of infertility: primary and secondary. Perhaps because fertility has long been considered exclusively a woman's issue, the diagnosis of primary or secondary infertility is dependent on the past and current reproductive status of the woman in the couple, rather than that of the man. In couples where the woman has never been pregnant the diagnosis would be *primary infertility*. This is the case even if the male partner has fathered a pregnancy previously. If the woman is able to achieve a pregnancy but experiences recurring miscarriages, the diagnosis is likely to be *subfertility*.

If, however, the woman has been pregnant in the past and either terminated the pregnancy or carried it to term, and she is now unable either to become pregnant again or to maintain a viable pregnancy, the couple's diagnosis would be *secondary infertility*. So the medical status of the male partner, while relevant in terms of the treatment of infertility, is not a factor in determining whether the couple are considered to have primary or secondary infertility.

It would be inaccurate and misleading, however, to think of infertility as only a medical condition. It is also a social condition. In a world where most women and men have been socialized to believe that they will one day become parents, a world where the ability to procreate is highly valued, being infertile carries a considerable set of implications. Not only are relationships with spouses, friends, and family members affected, so too are career options, and the availability of other satisfying and socially acceptable role options. Within the fertile world it can be very isolating and painful to be living as an infertile person or couple.

Infertility also has psychological implications. This does not in any way mean that there are psychological causes for infertility. Quite the contrary. Thirty to forty years ago, when 50 percent of all fertility problems could not be explained medically, it was assumed that psychological issues could cause a couple's infertility. As medical science and technology improved, however, so too did the ability of physicians to diagnose accurately the source of reproductive difficulties. Today only 5 to 10 percent of fertility problems remain undiagnosed (McShane 1997). Commonly referred to as "unexplained infertility," this inability of science even to provide answers as to the cause of their infertility often is one of the most challenging situations infertile couples face. Without answers or explanations, couples find it very difficult to make informed treatment decisions, and to know when they've done enough in their efforts to produce a child.

Although psychological problems are not the cause of infertility, there can be no doubt that infertility affects people psychologically. Being unable to produce a child who shares your genetic history and reflects the characteristics you love most about your partner is one of the saddest experiences in life. It is an experience that can challenge your most fundamental values and spiritual beliefs—about yourself, your relationship, the purpose of your life, and your God. It is an experience that affects how your value yourself and the way you feel about you body. Not being able to produce a child challenges your beliefs about the importance of family and genetic continuity. Moreover, trying to produce a child through the long and uncertain process of medical investigations and treatments (a process with no guarantee of a successful outcome) is one of the most stressful experiences one can have in life.

How Common Is Infertility?

Estimates vary on the prevalence of infertility because they are usually based on the statistics of those who seek medical assistance. Given this fact, it is difficult to accurately determine how common infertility is. Infertility affects an estimated 10 to 12 percent of American couples of reproductive age. In the United States alone, approximately 5.3 million couples are infertile (Corson 1999; McShane 1997). This means that one in six couples who try to have children experience problems with their fertility. Of those, it is estimated that more than half seek medical assistance and pursue some form of treatment.

Are Fertility Problems on the Rise?

This is a difficult question to answer because statistics are not available on infertile people who don't seek medical assistance. Also, there are more treatment options available today than there were thirty years ago. Since the early 1980s the number of clinics in the United States offering assisted reproductive technology has grown from 5 to 315 as of 1997. In Canada there are currently 23 fertility clinics providing these services. Furthermore, with fewer babies available for adoption, more couples may be seeking treatment now than in the past, thereby escalating the figures.

That being said, there has been some evidence that environmental toxins, chemicals and hormones in our foods, and other factors may be implicated in increasing the prevalence of fertility difficulties. These remain to be confirmed. What has changed, however, is the age when women and men begin trying to start their families. In the 1950s and 1960s the average age for a first pregnancy was the early twenties for women and the mid-twenties for men. Thirty was the recommended upper limit for couples having children—especially first children—and, in fact, pregnancies in women over thirty were considered high risk by medical professionals. Today over one third of all first births are to women over thirty. Close to 18 percent of all first births are to women over thirty-five. Because of the advancements in reproductive technologies it is not uncommon for couples to pursue a first pregnancy in their forties—something that would have been unheard of thirty years ago.

Changes in endocrine functioning that can negatively affect fertility have been documented for women beginning in the mid-thirties. As a woman's age increases, so too does the risk of spontaneous miscarriage and congenital abnormalities. For example, women over forty are five times as likely to miscarry as women between thirty and thirty-five. There have been indications that increasing age can be associated with decreased fertility for men as well. Certainly, advanced age is associated with more problems conceiving and carrying a pregnancy to term. This does not mean, however, that infertility is a problem only for those who wait until their thirties or forties to start their families.

Who Is Affected?

Infertility is a relatively indiscriminate affliction. It is a condition that strikes people in all racial and ethnic groups, crosses all socioeconomic classes, and affects both women and men relatively equally.

Women can have problems with their hormones; the quality of their eggs; the transfer of the sperm, egg, or embryo through the fallopian tubes; or the implantation of the embryo in the uterine lining. Female factor issues account for approximately 35 to 40 percent of fertility problems. Men can have difficulty with the quality of their semen in terms of count (numbers of sperm), morphology (shape/formation), or motility (percentage of sperm that are moving). They can also have obstructions that prevent the sperm from being released, or abnormalities that prevent the sperm from functioning effectively. Male factor issues account for about 30 to 35 percent of known fertility problems. An estimated 15 to 25 percent of fertility problems include some combination of both male and female factor issues, while 10 percent remain undiagnosed.

Although fertility declines with age, the inability to become pregnant or to maintain a pregnancy happens to individuals and couples at all stages of their reproductive lifespan. Those who attend fertility clinics generally tend to be older, often in their thirties and forties. There are, however, men and women in their twenties who also struggle with infertility. Younger couples frequently spend more time with general practitioners and gynecologists, before being referred to a clinic that specializes in treating infertility.

Is There a Typical Infertile Couple?

People come to the decision to start a family in different ways and at different times in their lives. As such, there really isn't a "typical" infertile couple. There are, however, some common ways couples arrive at the point in their lives where their fertility takes on critical importance. Three typical scenarios are described below.

People Who Always Wanted Children

About half of those who experience infertility say they have always known they wanted children. For them, having a family and being a parent has always been an important life goal. For many of these women and men, the decision to start a family was based on a feeling that they had reached the "right time" in their lives and relationships to become parents. Most had expectations of the age and what circumstances under which they wanted to start having children—expectations often based on their experiences of growing up in their own families.

For example, like many women, Karen always pictured herself as a mother. She recalls dressing her cat up in dolls' clothes and parading it around the neighborhood in a baby stroller. When she and Mike met, they talked about children and were agreed that they didn't want to wait too long to start their family. They wanted to be young when their kids were young and expected that by the time they reached their fifties, they'd be finished with the child-rearing part of their lives. They married in their mid-twenties, and within a couple of years started trying to have a baby.

When their initial efforts to produce a child didn't result in a pregnancy they were both surprised. Both came from large families. Neither had anticipated having any difficulty with their fertility. When they sought medical advice their physician told them not to worry, that they were young and a pregnancy just takes time. They were sent home with the advice to "relax" and "keep trying." It was another three years before a urologist confirmed that Mike was unable to produce sperm, most likely because of a groin injury he had sustained when playing junior hockey in his early teens.

The timetable for other couples may begin a bit later: after they establish their careers, or once they settle down with someone with whom they want to have children. For these couples it has never been an issue of *if* they are going to have children, only an issue of *when*. When they find out that they might not be able to have kids, their vision of their future is profoundly challenged.

People Who Thought They Would Never Want Children

These days many couples decide to become parents a bit later in their lives. They may have thought that having kids was something they'd consider in the future, or they may not have anticipated wanting children. A lot of women and men who experience infertility had not previously envisioned themselves as parents but, at some point in their lives, usually in their thirties or forties, their priorities started to shift and having children became important.

For women this shift usually occurs at some time in their thirties. It is not uncommon for women in their thirties who had thought they'd never want children to find their priorities and values changing. Given the very real biological limitations on women's fertility, the desire to have children often becomes more pressing for women at this stage of life. The biological clock begins to tick louder and they feel that they're running out of time.

Men seem to be on a somewhat different track developmentally. They don't face the same time limits on their fertility and therefore are not as pressured by the passage of time. For men who had never felt driven to have children, it is often in their early to mid-forties that fatherhood becomes important. It is common at this stage in a man's life to slow down enough to consider the future. Men often start to think about their own mortality and may find themselves, for the first time in their lives, thinking about becoming fathers.

Brad and Nancy are a good example of this type of infertile couple. In his twenties, Brad never thought much about having kids. With his education and a career to pursue, as well as an itch for traveling, having children was a nonissue. He later recalled that it crossed his mind at times, when a close friend or family member had a baby. But he couldn't really imagine himself as a parent, nor even conceive of how parenthood might fit into his life.

Similarly, his partner Nancy was quite convinced when they met that she didn't have a maternal bone in her entire body. She had watched her friends lose their freedom and become obsessively focused on formulas, diapers, and toilet training, and she was adamant that that wasn't going to happen to her. Both she and Brad couldn't figure out what all the fuss was about. They enjoyed their nieces and nephews, and the company of some of their friends who had children—the ones who could still talk about something other than their kids—but they felt no desire to become parents themselves. Nancy even recalled being curious enough about the transformation of some of her friends who had children to ask them what they got out of the experience? Why were they willing to give up so much to become parents. However, their answers did not seem convincing enough to make her want to change places with them. Having kids just wasn't for her!

Or so she thought, until something shifted. When she was thirty-five Nancy got to the point in her career where she felt that she'd really established herself. She found herself wondering "what's next?" Around the time of her thirty-fifth birthday she looked toward the future and wondered, "Is this all there is—will the next thirty or forty years just be more of the same?" She felt having children together was the next step she and Brad needed to take if they were going to continue to grow as a couple. Much to her surprise, having kids was starting to feel like something she wanted, and *needed*, to do.

On the other hand, at the age of thirty-seven Brad was just starting to hit his stride in his career. He was putting in long days and feeling a lot of pressure to establish a solid financial base so that he could afford to do the things he loved to do. At times, he even entertained the idea of retiring early. He *liked* his life and relationship with Nancy just the way they were. He wasn't ready to have children, but after a year of arguments and some serious soul-searching, he agreed to take the leap into parenthood. Like many couples in their mid- to late thirties, Nancy and Brad assumed they still had time and were surprised when they had difficulty becoming pregnant.

Couples in Remarriages

For another group of infertile men and women, those who find themselves in second or third marriages or whose partners have previously been married, the decision to start a family is frequently even more complex. A good example would be Dayna, thirty-four, and Jim, fifty-two. Jim had been married previously and had two grown children. His experience of parenting had not been especially positive. Although he currently had good relationships with his kids, he definitely did not want to have any more children. He'd had a vasectomy shortly after his second child was born, which Dayna had known about when they married. Initially, she was content with the idea of not having children, but as time went by she began to feel as if she was missing out on something important.

She and Jim struggled with the issue for a couple of years, and for a short period of time they even separated over it. Eventually Jim decided that he didn't want to be with anyone but Dayna, and if having kids was that important to her, then it really wasn't fair of him to deprive her of the experience. So, at the point in life when most of his friends were starting to plan their retirement, Jim had to rework his self-image and future goals to include becoming a parent again with a new family.

For older men like Jim, having kids is developmentally off schedule. The idea usually requires a reworking of current and future priorities. It requires the belief that *this* time around parenting will be a more positive experience than it was the first time. It may require a vasectomy reversal or high-tech fertility treatment. It may also mean making a decision to create and raise a child who is genetically related to the woman he loves but not to him, through the use of donor sperm.

For Whom Is Infertility Hardest?

For those who have always felt that having children was an important life goal, being unable to have a baby can shake their foundations and present an extremely challenging life crisis. Often their sense of masculinity or femininity is closely connected to their ability to procreate. Being infertile, then, strongly challenges their self-definition and self-worth. They may feel out of step with their friends and family members who are having children. Envisioning a life without children is especially difficult for these couples, making it very hard for them to give up their treatment efforts. Being parents is central to their self-definition and to their relationship. However, these couples often know that, one way or another, they will become parents. They'd love to have their own biological children, but, ultimately, being parents is their most important goal. As painful as it is not to be able to have their own children, sometimes such couples find it easier to move on to other parenting options. In my experience, if their treatment efforts are not successful, they rarely elect to remain childless.

Those who had never anticipated wanting children also find the experience of being unable to produce a child very painful. No matter what path people take in deciding they want to have children, once they start trying, their desire intensifies. In fact, couples who were initially ambivalent or equivocal about having children are often surprised at the importance having a child begins to assume in their lives. Many of these couples have been able to achieve most of what they had hoped for in their lives, and the fact that they are now unable to control something as important as their fertility is often very difficult to bear.

They frequently struggle with the belief that if they just tried hard enough they could "conquer the infertility beast," and most experience tremendous distress and frustration when their efforts aren't successful. This distress can be heightened when they are out of sync with their partners in terms of their desire to pursue or abandon treatment, given that having children wasn't a life goal they had originally set for themselves as a couple.

To their advantage, however, many of these couples can regain a sense of personal power and control in the pursuit of other parenting options if medical treatment fails to help them. Those who choose to remain childless often find ways to redirect their energies toward other satisfying goals.

How Do People Cope?

For any couple faced with infertility, the road ahead is not an easy one. The quest to produce a child can become all-consuming. People commonly find themselves experiencing a wide range of intense emotions, from fear to anger to desperation, as they try to cope both with the monthly reminders that their bodies have failed them, and with the pain, invasiveness, and uncertainty of medical testing and treatments. (See chapter 2 for information about the most common diagnostic and treatment procedures.)

In a way, being unable to produce a child is similar to other important losses in life. It's like a death—and people often respond as they would to a death, initially with surprise and denial, followed by periods of intense anger, feelings of guilt and unworthiness, sadness and depression, and grief.

But infertility is also different from most other losses in life. Because it is the loss of potential life, the loss of a dream and a life goal, it is largely invisible. This fact alone makes it very difficult for many couples who are struggling with infertility to get the support and understanding they need from others.

Then, too, the experience of being unable to produce a child is unique in that it can go on for many years without resolution. Couples can spend years trying to find solutions to their fertility problems, all that time living in the space between being infertile and being parents—not yet pregnant but ever hopeful that medical science will help them to have a child. The possibility that their infertility will be permanent is always there, but so too is the possibility that eventually they'll become parents. This uncertainty makes it very hard for couples to get on with their lives, because they really can't plan for the future. A future that includes parenthood looks quite different than a future without children.

So, unlike concrete and visible losses, infertility is invisible. Also, unlike other significant losses, such as the loss of a job or the death of a parent, it is not possible to predict how any individual or couple will react to their inability to produce a child. Although it is an experience shared by many men and women, each person's experience of infertility is highly personal.

Responses to infertility differ depending on each person's personality traits, beliefs about the meaning and importance of parenthood, their age, their relationship with their partner, and whether there are other available roles that can give their lives meaning. Reactions differ as a result of which partner is diagnosed with the fertility problem, and whether an explanation is ever found for the couple's inability to become pregnant or carry a pregnancy to term.

How people react to infertility, how they cope, and the ways in which they express their feelings also seem to differ by their sex. Consistent with the way women and men have been socialized, women are usually much more expressive of their feelings of sadness, grief, and loss over being unable to produce a child. This doesn't necessarily mean that becoming a parent is more important for a woman than it is for a man, or that being unable to produce a child is less painful for a man than for a woman. It simply means that women and men tend to express feelings and respond to distress in different ways. These differences are discussed at length in chapter 5, with suggestions that will help you and your partner begin to understand these differences and work with them, making infertility for both of you easier to cope with.

Another gender difference worth noting here is that, in almost all cases, it is the woman who takes responsibility for initiating medical fertility investigations and treatments, so don't be surprised if this is the case in your relationship. Maybe it's because throughout their lives women tend to become more involved with medical practitioners. Or perhaps it is because fertility and infertility are socially viewed as women's issues. It is generally assumed that if a couple is having difficulty becoming pregnant it's the woman's fault. Couples often go along with this assumption. Whatever the reasons for the woman's taking the lead, this pattern usually continues throughout the treatment process. If treatment fails, however, and couples decide to pursue other parenting options, the pattern often shifts to more shared initiation.

Basic Strategies for Surviving Infertility

In some ways your experience of infertility may be similar to that of other infertile people. However, although this is a fairly common experience, your infertility is also unique to you. As you read the stories and suggestions throughout this book, it will be important for you to recognize the personal nature of your experience. You will see yourself and your partner in some of these examples, but not in others. You also may find some of the strategies and suggestions more useful than others, so be selective. How you cope with your infertility and make decisions about your treatment and parenting options must be in line with what works best for you and for your partner. With that in mind, let's look at some overall guidelines or general strategies that might help the two of you to deal with the stresses and strains of infertility.

Strategy Number One: Don't Assume You Have Control

Until recently, like most people you probably assumed that your fertility was under your control. Unless you were born with a physical problem, or experienced a specific trauma to your reproductive organs when you were younger, you probably grew up believing that, if and when you were ready, you'd be able to start a family.

This isn't surprising. The desire to procreate is one of humankind's strongest instincts. From the time you were very young you were taught that having children is the natural, normal thing to do. Overall, you were probably careful to avoid an accidental pregnancy. Once you reached a certain age, especially if you were married, others most likely asked you when you were going to start your family. If you didn't want children before now, especially if you are a woman, you might have wondered if you were normal.

Given this type of socialization, when you finally stopped using contraception it's likely that you expected to become pregnant within a few months. When it didn't happen right away, you were probably quite surprised. This is the most common initial reaction to infertility. Even women who have had problems with their periods, or men who have had a groin injury or undescended testicles in childhood, are still surprised when their efforts to produce a child are unsuccessful. As Dorothy, a thirty-two-year old dietitian, says in the quote below, not being able to control your fertility can come as quite a shock:

> *I'm really not a control freak, but this was one area of my life that I thought I'd always have control over. You know, I was always very careful when I was younger about not getting pregnant. And I was on the pill for about five years before we started trying to have a baby . . . five years when I thought I was in control of my fertility. When I didn't get pregnant it came as quite a shock.*

The belief that people have control over their fertility is widely supported socially as well. Most likely, since you've been trying to get pregnant you've been repeatedly confronted with others' advice to "just relax," "take a holiday," or "adopt a child—then you'll probably get pregnant." Steve, a thirty-eight-year-old man who, with his partner, Michele, struggled for six years with unexplained infertility, explains it this way:

> Lots of people gave us advice: . . . "Maybe you're not doing it right," "Have a glass of wine or two before you go to bed," "Relax," "Try standing on your head after sex." Even doctors told us, "You're trying too hard. Relax . . . it'll happen eventually."

The implication is that either you're trying "too hard" or not trying "hard enough" to become pregnant, and that somehow you are blocking your fertility.

The belief that your fertility is under your control is a natural assumption. However, it can get you into a lot of trouble as you try to cope with infertility and make informed treatment decisions. You may find yourself planning your treatment cycles for the times in your life or career when you're less stressed, not just because it will make it easier to cope, but because you believe your chances of success will be better if you're more relaxed. Or, if you're like many people, you may hold yourself accountable when a particular treatment cycle fails: you weren't relaxed enough, you exerted yourself too much, you didn't have a positive attitude, you didn't eat the right foods or think the right thoughts. The list is endless, but the outcome is the same: you feel as though it's your fault that you're not pregnant.

In dealing with infertility, one of the hardest things to come to terms with is that you really don't have control over the outcome. Fertility is a biological process involving a complex set of hormonal and physiological reactions and the right anatomical conditions. You can be in excellent health and physical condition, and you can manage your stress in very healthy and productive ways. Certainly, good nutrition, exercise, and a positive attitude can be enormously helpful in managing the stress of treatment and the distress of being unable to produce a child. However, try as you might, you can't control your fertility. Coming to terms with this reality—learning to accept the things you don't have control of and taking control over the things you do—is one of the most important things you can do to survive.

Strategy Number Two: Try Not to Panic

When you don't get pregnant right away, it is important not to panic. It is not unusual for couples to have twelve months of regular unprotected intercourse to secure a viable first pregnancy. This may be hard to believe especially since most of us recall the warnings we heard when we were teenagers to be careful about having sex because "you only have to do it once to get pregnant." And since you've been trying to become pregnant, you've probably heard countless people say that their partner just has to look at them a certain way and—bang—they get pregnant, or that they planned the birth of their children to the day or month.

The truth is that getting pregnant takes time. First, there are only a few days in any menstrual cycle when a pregnancy can occur. One egg is usually released during each menstrual cycle. The egg, or oocyte, as it is commonly called in medical terms, is only capable of being fertilized by the sperm within the first eighteen to twenty-four hours after it is released. With approximately thirteen cycles a year, assuming that the woman is on a regular twenty-eight-day cycle (which many women are not), that means there are only about twenty-six days a year when conception is even possible.

Also, the average chance of conceiving in a month for couples having regular intercourse throughout the menstrual cycle, meaning approximately three times per week, is only about 20 percent per cycle when the woman is less than thirty-five years of age. As the age of the woman increases beyond thirty-five years, the spontaneous conception rate is estimated to decrease each year. Once a woman is forty years or older, the per cycle rate of conception is only 5 percent.

It is also important to remember that the process of conception is very complex. That is why even the most advanced reproductive technologies are not always successful. When you think about everything that has to happen—sperm meeting egg; sperm penetrating egg; egg dividing into an eight-celled embryo; embryo traveling down the fallopian tube, breaking out of its protective outer covering (the *zona pellucida*), and implanting in the uterine wall—it is quite amazing that anyone ever becomes pregnant. Finally, the risk of miscarriage also increases markedly with age from less than 12 percent for women under thirty-five to approximately 34 percent for women between forty and forty-four years. Clearly, for many couples, achieving a viable pregnancy takes time.

So, whether you're at the beginning of the process of dealing with infertility, or you're currently undergoing a number of medicated or unmedicated intrauterine insemination cycles, try not to panic if you don't become pregnant right away. If you and your partner have fairly normal reproductive histories, and the medical tests haven't turned up any specific problems, it may just be a matter of time.

If you're pursuing some of the more advanced interventions, also try to remember that, however amazing these technologies are, intervening in the creation of life is far from an exact science. With each treatment cycle the physicians and laboratory specialists may learn more about your particular situation and be more able to tailor their recommendations to your unique needs.

Strategy Number Three: Within Reason, Be Patient

It is important to be patient within reason—especially in the beginning. You may have been on birth control pills for an extended period of time and it may take a while for your endocrine system to get back to its own rhythm. Or, when you look back at the preceding months spent trying to conceive you may realize that there really weren't that many times when you had intercourse while you were likely to be ovulating.

If you're under thirty, you've had no previous conditions that might affect reproduction (e.g., in women, endometriosis, pelvic inflammatory disease, very irregular menstrual cycles, or abdominal surgery, in men, undescended testicles, a groin injury, mumps during adolescence, or working with or near toxic substances, etc.), and neither of your families has a history of fertility problems such as premature menopause or severe male factor infertility, you can probably afford to wait about twelve months before assuming that something is wrong. If, however, you're over thirty, you or your partner has a history of any of the problems listed above, or there is a family history of fertility problems, you might consider taking action sooner.

Patience is also important when you're undergoing treatments. As I said earlier, once you decide you want to have children and realize you're having trouble doing so, your sense of urgency increases. You may feel as though the clock is ticking and you're very anxious to do whatever it's going to take to get this fixed. It seems to take forever to get appointments for medical consultations and to arrange treatment cycles.

If you had expected to have your first child and to be finished with having kids by a particular age you may already feel like you're off schedule. And if you hear about one more friend or family member who is pregnant, you feel as is you might scream. Worse yet, you've heard about how women over thirty-five can have more difficulty getting pregnant—much less women over forty—and you're afraid you're going to be one of those women. As thirty-nine-year-old

Paula says below, it's as if you're in a race with a biological or social clock, and you feel like you're losing:

I always thought I'd be a mother by the time I was thirty. But then I was busy with other things and I hadn't met anyone whom I really wanted to have kids with . . . and I wasn't ready to do this on my own. Then I met Jack, and it took some time to work out our relationship. So the time just seemed to fly by and before I knew it I was thirty-seven and I thought, yikes, I always wanted at least two kids and I'm running out of time.

In fact, there is nothing magical about the ages of thirty-five and forty. It is not as if a switch is flipped after these birthdays, causing your fertility to take a nosedive. The reality is that for most women, and for men too, minor, usually imperceptible hormonal changes begin in the thirties and continue throughout the forties. These changes can affect fertility over time, but they are rarely dramatic at any one point in time. So a person's fertility at age forty is usually not dramatically different than his or her fertility at age thirty-nine. As hard as it can be, do your best to be patient.

Strategy Number Four: Be Assertive

When you first realize you are having difficulty becoming pregnant and you decide to consult a physician before the usual twelve months are up, don't be surprised if you are told to go home and keep trying. This is pretty standard medical advice, especially when the woman in the couple is under thirty-five years of age. When the woman is over thirty-five, fertility specialists characteristically recommend investigations after six months of trying, although some family doctors still make their recommendations using the twelve-month definition of infertility.

It is also important to know that, in cases of impaired fertility, medical investigations and treatments can take months or even years before an answer is found. Despite the advancements in reproductive technologies, is not unusual for couples to spend several years from the time they start trying to have a family to the time they achieve a pregnancy or decide to terminate medical treatment. When you are facing very real biological limitations on your fertility, it may well pay to be assertive about trying to find answers and solutions. After going through years of medical investigations and treatments, many of the infertile men and women I've worked with have said that one of their biggest regrets is that they weren't more assertive about having their concerns addressed and their needs met when they first realized that their fertility might be a problem. Diana's words reflect this sense of regret:

> You know, looking back now I just wish we'd got on with it sooner. Not with starting to have kids—we weren't ready yet—but once we started and it wasn't happening, I just wish we'd pushed a little harder to get the answers. In the long run we'd have ended up where we are now, but it wouldn't have taken so long. We wouldn't have spent so many years in limbo—with our entire lives on hold.

Being assertive, however, is often easier said than done—especially when you're dealing with the medical profession. Most of us have learned to defer to our doctors' recommendations. If our physician tells us to take a particular pill or wait a few more months before starting a specific treatment, it can be very difficult to challenge his or her knowledge and advice, especially when we're already feeling vulnerable and when they're the experts in their field. When we walk into a physician's office we become patients, and making demands is not consistent with the patient's role.

Also, many couples are afraid to ask questions or challenge the recommendations of their specialists, for fear of being seen as difficult or noncompliant patients. The words of Bob, a twenty-nine-year-old salesman, capture these sentiments:

> They're the experts, the one's who are supposed to know best. And when you finally get to see these guys, even if you don't agree with what they're recommending, it's really hard to say, "No, we'd rather not do that," or "We've been reading up on this and we think we'd rather do this treatment instead."
> There are lots more couples just like you waiting to take your place. It's amazing how easy it is to let someone with authority tell you this is what you need to be doing with your body and with your life and with your spirit.

At all stages of the medical treatment process it is important to find some balance between being assertive about your needs and desires, and being receptive to your physician's advice. One of the best ways to do this is to maintain an open and ongoing dialogue between you and your partner about what you both feel needs to happen and when, and about what you both can handle. It is also helpful not to place the entire burden of responsibility for your treatment decisions on your physician.

Strategy Number Five: Be an Informed Consumer

Fertility diagnosis and treatment is a world unto itself, and when you enter into this world you may feel like Alice falling through the looking glass. The group of physicians and researchers in this medical specialty, known as reproductive endocrinology, focus exclusively on fertility problems. Since the birth of the first test-tube baby, Louise Brown, in 1978, the treatment of infertility has become an industry that brings in 2 billion dollars a year. In the past ten years alone, scientists have literally revolutionized the treatment of male factor infertility by learning how to extract sperm from the testicles of previously infertile men, and by finding methods to guide individual sperm into the eggs of their partners.

The technological advancements are remarkable and provide new hope for many infertile couples. But many of these advancements are also controversial. You may find yourselves confronting some very difficult moral and ethical dilemmas as you undergo treatment, such as whether to selectively reduce a multiple pregnancy if you end up expecting more than two babies as a result of in vitro fertilization or hormone therapy.

These difficulties are also compounded by the fact that many treatments are relatively new and, as such, accurate success rates are not available for the full range of infertile patients who have attempted these treatments. The long-term consequences of some of the more powerful hormonal medications and complex treatment options also remain to be determined, both in terns of the social and health implications for the couple as well as the child or children they produce. These realities can make informed decision making extremely difficult.

It is impossible for a lay person to become well versed in all the available diagnostic procedures, medications, and treatment options. However, you are well advised to become as informed a consumer as possible while coping with your fertility difficulties and making treatment decisions. In the words of Cindy, a woman who spent five years undergoing the full range of fertility treatments:

> I would really advise people to try to get as much information as they can, and to ask lots of questions. A lot of things are kind of vague and physicians don't usually have a lot of time. So it's up to you. As a couple you've got to do the digging and the researching—it's up to you to find out what questions need to be asked.

See chapter 2 for some of the more common tests, terminology, and interventions. There are also some excellent resources listed at the back of this book that clearly describe the treatment procedures, the various side effects, and the potential risks.

Strategy Number Six: Don't Blame Yourself or Your Partner

One of the most common reactions when something negative happens in life is to wonder what you did, or didn't do, to cause it. Infertility is no exception. Women and men who find they are unable to produce a child either on their own, or with medical assistance, frequently blame themselves. This is especially the case for the member of the couple who is found to have the fertility impairment, but even those who don't have an identifiable problem often wonder what they did to deserve their infertility. Women particularly tend to blame themselves, even when their partner has been diagnosed with a male factor fertility problem.

Whatever your situation, you may well find yourself rummaging through your history, looking for some explanation for your infertility. Perhaps you terminated a pregnancy in the past, or relinquished a child for adoption; maybe you were sexually active before meeting your partner, or perhaps you've had an extramarital affair. You may be worrying that one of your past actions has caused your current infertility problem. You may beat yourself up for not trying to start a family earlier, or for choosing a partner who isn't fertile.

Although such thoughts are common, they aren't especially helpful for coping with infertility. They only make you feel worse about yourself or your partner, and although your past may contain things that you regret, they probably didn't cause your fertility problems. Women who have fertility problems when they're in their thirties may well have encountered the same problems had they tried to become pregnant earlier. And men whose sperm counts aren't high now may never have had high counts.

Regrets are futile and so is blame. The decisions you made in the past are past, and they were made at a different time in your life. Energy wasted on what was or what might have been can be much better used for coping with your current reality and in trying to make satisfying life, parenting, and treatment decisions. As Paul, a thirty-four-year-old infertile artist, aptly stated:

*You don't want to be stressing yourself out and blaming
yourself or your partner for things you can't control. As lousy
as it is, just accept the situation and go on with what you
think is the best thing to do next. It's all you can do.*

Strategy Number Seven: Don't Expect This to Make Sense

One of the hardest things to come to terms with is the injustice of the situation. Most people struggling with infertility are decent folk who have done their best to lead responsible lives. Many have really labored over the decision about whether to bring a child into the world, and they have done their best to ensure that they have a solid relationship and adequate economic resources in place to meet the needs of a child.

The injustice of infertility becomes particularly difficult to cope with when you hear stories about parents who abandon or abuse their children, or when you read about newborns with fetal alcohol syndrome or babies born to mothers who are drug addicts. Friends complain about their children and make envious comments about how lucky you are because you can come and go as you please and sleep late on the weekends. They take parenthood for granted, having absolutely no idea how much you'd love to be in their shoes. This frustration is apparent in the words of Maggie, a thirty-three-year-old writer diagnosed with premature ovarian failure:

*I resent these women at the grocery store, when I see them in
line—the way they yank their kids around and shout at them
and scold them. It's like, "God, if they could only walk in our
shoes for a while, and let every parent learn to appreciate their
child all over again. If only they knew how lucky they are."*

If you're like most infertile couples, you believe you'd make good parents, and you can't understand why you and your partner are being denied something so important, something others take for granted or don't seem to deserve. It doesn't seem fair and no matter how hard you try, you just can't make sense out of it. You may ask yourself if you're being tested, thinking that maybe you just have to prove how important having children is for you.

There are no answers. Infertility isn't fair. You don't deserve to be infertile, and you and your partner haven't been singled out for this particularly difficult challenge because of something you did, or didn't do, in your lives. It's like being dealt a bad hand—one you just have to play. One infertile woman's words say it best:

> *Infertility is just something that life gives you . . . like some*
> *people get cancer, or are in a bad accident, or have health*
> *problems, or a disability, or children who don't turn out well.*
> *Everybody has something they have to deal with in life.*
> *Infertility is just one of those things and by chance it*
> *happened to us. There's no point in trying to understand why;*
> *we just have to deal with it.*

The information in the following chapters is meant to help you do just that.

2

Traversing the Medical Minefield

Depending on whether you begin you medical investigations with a general practitioner, a gynecologist, or an infertility specialist (also known as a reproductive endocrinologist), the course of medical investigations and the treatment options that are recommended to you may differ. In any case, beginning the process of diagnosis and treatment can be a bit daunting. You may find yourselves wondering why particular tests are ordered, what the results mean, and the reasons certain treatments are recommended while others are not. You may also find the medical terminology difficult to understand and sometimes even a bit disparaging (e.g., "hostile" cervical mucus).

There are some standard tests that, according to the American Society for Reproductive Medicine's practice committee (2000), should be included in the optimal medical fertility evaluation. Depending on the results of these diagnostic assessments specific treatment options will normally be recommended. These evaluations and treatments are briefly described below. Common tests and terminology are also defined, as are some of the emotional issues associated with specific investigations and treatment options.

The information below is meant to be an overview to help prepare you for what might lie ahead as you work your way through what, at times, can feel a bit like a medical minefield. There are many comprehensive resources that explain the medical management of fertility problems, and this chapter is not meant to replace them. The information in this chapter is also not intended to be a substitute for a discussion about your individual circumstances with your health care provider. If you want to learn more about your particular diagnosis, or about certain tests or treatments that are being recommended by your physician, I encourage you to refer to the excellent resources listed at the back of this book. In particular, *Conquering Infertility: A Guide for Couples*, by Stephen Corson (1999), provides detailed diagnostic and treatment information in very understandable language.

The Initial Medical Workup

When you first begin fertility investigations your physician will assess your medical history and that of your partner in an attempt to determine the possible reasons you haven't been able to get pregnant. A thorough evaluation is critical in ensuring a prompt and accurate diagnosis, and in providing your physician with the necessary information upon which to base his or her treatment recommendations. Infertility is a couple's issue. Both partners need to attend the appointment and both will necessarily be involved in the medical investigations. The workup usually begins with a number of basic questions, either in the form of a questionnaire or an interview. Some of these questions may seem odd to you and you might wonder what they have to do with your fertility, but the answers can help to provide important clues to why you might be having difficulty becoming pregnant. So let's take a look at what you'll need to be prepared to discuss during the initial medical workup. If you are a man, this includes information on:

- your general state of health, including current medications (prescription and naturopathic) and chronic illnesses

- the extent and nature of your physical activities

- your social habits, including smoking, use of recreational drugs, alcohol consumption, use of steroids, etc.

- symptoms of possible endocrine (hormone) changes—fatigue, diabetes-related symptoms, headaches, visual changes

- previous injuries to your testicles or groin area, spinal cord, or head

- any pregnancies you've fathered in the past and if so, when they occurred, and the outcome of the pregnancies

- genetic abnormalities, or any problems at birth such as undescended testicles

- previous surgeries on the testicles, hernias, or vasectomy reversal

- treatments for cancer with radiation or chemotherapy

- exposure (usually work-related) to chemicals, radiation, toxins, or extremes of heat or cold

- infectious diseases including mumps and sexually transmitted infections

- sexual history and current behavior—frequency and adequacy of erection and ejaculation; whether orgasm occurs during intercourse; frequency of intercourse

The information your physician requires to assess the female partner is similar in many ways, but of course considerable emphasis is placed on the woman's menstrual and reproductive history. So, if you are a woman you will likely be asked about:

- when you started menstruating

- the regularity, timing, and duration of your periods, whether these have recently changed, and if so in what way

- past pregnancies, their outcome, and any associated complications

- your history and methods of birth control

- your current sexual frequency

- the length of time you have been trying to conceive

- any previous diagnosis of pelvic inflammatory disease (PID), chlamydia, or a sexually transmitted disease (e.g., gonorrhea)

- your medical and surgical history, previous hospitalizations, serious illness or injuries, and childhood disorders

- abnormal pap smears and subsequent treatments

- allergies and current medications

- your current level of health and fitness

- your alcohol consumption, smoking, and use of recreational drugs

- symptoms of thyroid disease, pelvic or abdominal pain, or painful intercourse

- current physical or psychological conditions (e.g., depression)

- a family history of reproductive failure, birth defects, or mental retardation

It is estimated that about 5 percent of fertility problems are the result of sexual difficulties, and, as noted in chapter 1, the window of fertility during each menstrual cycle is relatively small. Because the timing of intercourse is so crucial, you and your partner will need to be prepared to discuss with the health-care provider whether and when you have sexual relations, how often, and whether the man has ejaculation during intercourse.

All of this information is important in the initial diagnosis of your fertility problem. However, because many of the questions focus on what for most of us is a very private part of our lives, you may find it difficult to answer them openly. Perhaps you haven't already shared some of this information with your partner, or maybe in your culture these issues aren't addressed openly, even between partners. In these cases you might ask to be interviewed separately, or you might request to be able to put your answers in writing rather than having to respond verbally. You may also find some of the suggestions in chapter 4 helpful in coping with the stresses throughout this and subsequent parts of your medical investigations and treatments.

Evaluation of the Man

Compared to that of women, men's physical role in the reproductive process is relatively uncomplicated. It follows, then, that the extent of diagnostic testing for men is also more limited. In essence, it comes down to assessing the adequate production and delivery of sperm. Once it has been determined in your initial medical workup that you are having regular intercourse and are not experiencing problems with your sexual functioning, such as premature or retrograde ejaculation, the medical investigation of your fertility will likely involve: a physical examination, semen analysis, and in some cases laboratory testing.

The Physical Examination

Your family physician will probably have conducted a complete general examination prior to referring you for more specialized investigations. The examination conducted by your urologist or fertility specialist will focus more specifically on your genitals—your penis, urethra, scrotum, and testes. This examination will help to rule out common causes of male factor fertility problems: abnormalities in the testicles, the presence of a *varicocele* or the absence of the vas deferens, a condition that occurs in men who may carry the cystic fibrosis gene. The condition of the prostate will also be assessed through a rectal examination.

Semen Analysis

In any fertility investigation, whether or not a problem is identified in the female partner, it is important that the male partner's sperm be analyzed. Poor semen quality accounts for an estimated 30 to 40 percent of all fertility problems (Corson 1999). Sperm problems can be caused by previous injury, congenital abnormalities, illness, chemotherapy and radiation, drug and alcohol use, a vasectomy, or an unsuccessful vasectomy reversal. Environmental issues such as exposure to toxins in the workplace have also been implicated as a cause of male infertility. In many cases, however, no clear cause can be found to explain why a man's sperm count is low or why his sperm aren't shaped properly or swimming correctly.

Sperm testing usually takes place two to five days after the man's last ejaculation. If abstinence prior to collection extends beyond five days, the sample quality may be compromised by the presence of too many dead sperm. The test requires that the man masturbate into a small sterile container, which is then taken within a specified time (usually one hour) to a laboratory for analysis. The sample needs to be kept close to body temperature during this time. Keeping the container next to the body or in your coat pocket during transport is usually adequate (Corson 1999). Many fertility clinics prefer that the sample be collected on site rather than at home, which can be a bit embarrassing and can present a challenge for some men. Needless to say, a clinical environment is not especially conducive to erotic thoughts and actions. On the other hand, the stress of having to produce the sample at a clinic may be offset by you not having to worry about keeping the sample warm while trying to get it to the laboratory within the required time.

Infertility is stressful enough, without the additional anxiety of having to produce a semen sample on demand. However, the semen analysis is the only way to assess the presence or absence of a male factor problem, so it's an unavoidable part of a thorough medical evaluation. If you find that you're pretty anxious about having to produce a sample, you might ask to have your partner accompany you. Many clinics also provide erotic magazines or movies, or allow you to bring in your own in order to make the collection a little easier. Clinic staff are aware that this situation can be stressful so they usually try to be sensitive and accommodating so that this process can be as comfortable for you as possible, under the circumstances.

Once your semen sample is received it will be analyzed. There are essentially two types of semen analysis: *standard analysis* and *specialized sperm screening*. A standard analysis provides your physician with basic information: whether there are sperm in the semen and how many (volume/amount), the percentage that are moving (motility), and the percentage that are normally shaped (morphology). According to the World Health Organization (1999) a normal semen analysis would have a volume of more than 2.0 ml (milliliters), a sperm count of greater than 20 million/ml, motility of over 50 percent, and morphology of more than 30 percent normal forms. If the semen analysis does not fall within normal parameters you may be asked to repeat the analysis after a couple of months to confirm the initial findings. If the second analysis confirms a problem with the sperm, specialized sperm screening may be recommended. You may also be referred to a urologist for further investigation and for confirmation of your treatment options.

Specialized sperm screening is less widely available and is a more complex and technically advanced approach to sperm testing that requires a well-equipped laboratory like those in specialized fertility centers. These tests enable your physician to determine with greater accuracy the characteristics assessed in a standard semen analysis, as well as the functional capabilities of the sperm—specifically, the particular processes involved in fertilization of the oocyte (egg). The results of the screening provide important information about the types of treatments that would, and would not, be likely to help you achieve a pregnancy.

Laboratory Testing

A relatively small number of reproductive problems in men are caused by hormonal problems such as decreased levels of testosterone, thyroid disease, or elevated prolactin levels (Corson 1999). When indicated, your doctor may recommend some blood tests as part of your fertility evaluation.

Evaluation of the Woman

Infertility testing and diagnosis of the woman is characteristically more complex. It involves assessing whether ovulation is occurring, the condition of the fallopian tubes and uterine cavity, and, in some cases, the cervix. There are a number of tests specific to making these determinations, each of which is discussed below. However, prior to ordering these tests your family doctor or specialist will conduct a thorough physical examination including a pelvic exam to identify any symptoms or signs that might suggest a specific cause for your inability to become pregnant. This information helps your physician determine which diagnostic tests to recommend next, given your particular situation.

The Physical Examination

The physical exam may include determination of your weight and body mass index (the degree to which your weight falls within a healthy range given your height). A body mass index number below twenty or above twenty-seven is associated with an increased risk of health problems for some individuals and may be related to or implicated in your problems with fertility. Your physician may also determine the size and tenderness of your thyroid gland, and he or she may ask whether you have been experiencing the secretion of any fluid from your nipples. A pelvic examination is conducted to assess the condition of the vagina, cervix, and uterus (ASRM 2000). This will likely be one of several pelvic examinations or procedures you experience during the course of your fertility investigations and treatments; if you feel uncomfortable during these examinations you might consider using some of the relaxation techniques suggested in chapter 4.

Assessing Ovulation

Ovulation is a critical component of the process of conception. Disorders of ovulation account for 20 to 25 percent of all fertility problems. The most common causes of ovulatory problems are hormonal imbalances, inherited predisposition, and advanced age (Keye 1999). Two aspects of ovulation are important in ensuring conception: the release of the egg and the quality of the egg. Your *menstrual history* is a good subjective indicator of whether you ovulate and how regularly you ovulate. Regular, relatively predictable periods that occur at predictable intervals are a sign of ovulation. Conversely, periods that are irregular in length and occur sporadically can be an indication of ovulatory problems, as can a history of irregular and heavy bleeding.

There are a number of other ways to determine whether you are ovulating. For example, you may be asked to record your *basal body temperature* (BBT). BBTs provide a relatively simple and inexpensive method for evaluating your ovulatory function (ASRM 2000). Your BBT is determined by taking your temperature every morning, before you get out of bed or become active, and charting your temperature using a special thermometer designed to indicate minor changes in temperature. An increase in temperature during the second half of the menstrual cycle is an indication that you have ovulated. Your physician may also ask you to indicate on your BBT chart the days you've had intercourse. This can help to indicate the intercourse frequency and timing that are most likely to result in a pregnancy.

Couples often rely on these temperature readings to time intercourse when they're trying to become pregnant. Unfortunately, BBTs tend not to be a very reliable indicator of *when* women will ovulate, only *if* they have ovulated. This being the case, basal body temperature readings are best considered a diagnostic tool, which most physicians recommend be taken for only a couple of months.

For an even more precise indicator of ovulation your doctor might recommend a blood test that measures your *serum progesterone levels*. Progesterone is the female hormone secreted by the *corpus luteum* (tissue formed in the ovary once the egg has been released) during the second half of the menstrual cycle. Progesterone helps prepare the *endometrium* (lining of the uterus) for implantation. When women ovulate, their progesterone levels rise. These tests are characteristically done in the last third of the menstrual cycle—seven to ten days before the last day of the cycle (e.g., day eighteen to twenty-one of a twenty-eight-day cycle; or day twenty-six to twenty-nine of a thirty-six-day cycle).

Ovulation predictor kits that detect the presence of the hormone LH (the hormone that triggers ovulation) in urine can also be used. However, they are expensive, and they may not be practical for women who have irregular periods, since they may not know the most likely day of ovulation or whether they are ovulating at all. As a result, ovulation predictor kits are best used for pinpointing the day of ovulation once a woman knows that she does ovulate. This can help in the timing of intercourse. But remember, ovulation predictor kits are not a good substitute for regular intercourse. Women have

been getting pregnant long before the invention of ovulation predictor kits, or even thermometers, for that matter.

A less frequently used indicator of ovulation is the *endometrial
biopsy*. The endometrium changes after ovulation in preparation for a
possible pregnancy. It is this lining that is cast off in the menstrual
blood during your period, if a pregnancy has not occurred. This procedure can be quite uncomfortable but fortunately it is over fairly
quickly. The physician inserts through the cervix a plastic or metal
object, which is then used to scrape a sample of tissue from the inside
of the uterus. The tissue is evaluated by a pathologist to determine if
the degree of development of the lining matches the day of your
menstrual cycle on which it was obtained. Again, you might find
some of the relaxation techniques discussed in chapter 4 to be helpful
during the endometrial biopsy.

If necessary your doctor may also recommend the mid-cycle
transvaginal ultrasound. This test involves a relatively painless procedure that can help to determine whether you are ovulating and can
provide information on the thickness and apparent adequacy of the
lining of your uterus.

It is also common for physicians to recommend a number of
standard blood tests as part of a basic infertility workup. Measuring
serum thyroid-stimulating hormone (TSH) and prolactin levels helps
to identify disorders of the thyroid gland and of prolactin production. Follicle-stimulating hormone (FSH) level evaluation and the
clomiphene citrate challenge test can provide important information
regarding the egg quality and responsiveness of the ovaries to hormones. Your doctor can use this information in determining the best
course of treatment if ovulatory functioning is causing your inability
to achieve a pregnancy (ASRM 2000).

Assessing the Fallopian Tubes and Uterus

If the less-invasive tests to determine ovulation show no indication of reasons you're not getting pregnant, and your physician has
been unable to detect a male factor problem, he or she will likely recommend more extensive assessments including an *hysterosalpingogram* (HSG), *sonohysterogram*, and perhaps a *laparoscopy* and
hysteroscopy. These tests will help to determine whether your fallopian tubes are open, or whether there is some other abnormality of
the uterine cavity or pelvis that might be preventing you from
becoming pregnant. Problems with the woman's tubes or pelvis are
implicated in 20 to 25 percent of fertility problems (Keye 1999). Tubal

blockage usually arises from some sort of infectious or inflammatory process in the pelvis such as a ruptured appendix, or may be a result of previous pelvic surgery, an episode of chlamydia or gonorrhea, endometriosis, or an intrauterine device (IUD) that allowed infection to travel up into the uterus and tubes.

The *hysterosalpingogram* is an X-ray of the fallopian tubes and uterus. It is a relatively noninvasive way to determine whether and where your tubes may be blocked as well as to define the size and shape of your uterus. However, the HSG is not a typical X-ray. It involves injection of a colorless liquid or "dye" into the opening of the cervix. While the dye is flowing through the uterus and tubes a series of pictures is taken.

Usually, this test is completed within a few minutes, but the procedure can be quite uncomfortable for some women, who report mild to severe cramping during or following the procedure. As well as relying on the relaxation techniques discussed in chapter 4, you may want to ask your physician to recommend a mild medication that you can take before the procedure, in order to reduce the possibility of abdominal cramping. Because of this discomfort, it can also be difficult to drive and go back to work immediately after the HSG, so you may want to consider having your partner or a friend drive you to and from the location for this procedure.

A recently developed procedure that can provide information similar to that of the HSG is known as a *sonohysterogram*. This method uses ultrasound instead of X-rays to see the uterus and fallopian tubes. This procedure sometimes fails to provide all the necessary information so an HSG may still be required.

Results of the HSG or sonohysterogram can provide critical diagnostic information. An obstruction of one or both fallopian tubes might indicate a problem for the sperm to reach the egg. Since most women don't ovulate on the same side each month, an obstruction in one tube would decrease your chances of conception in the months when ovulation occurs from the ovary on that side. If blockages are found in both tubes, the probability of conception without medical intervention would be nil.

Depending on what was learned from your initial workup, your physician may recommend a *laparoscopy*—a surgical procedure that allows direct visual assessment of the condition of a woman's ovaries, fallopian tubes, and uterus using a fiberoptic instrument. After a general anesthetic is administered, the physician makes a one-half-inch-long incision in the fold of skin at the belly button and another small incision just at the pubic hair line. Your abdomen is filled with carbon dioxide gas to make an air pocket for insertion of the small instruments. A small amount of this gas often remains under your diaphragm, which, surprisingly, may cause shoulder stiffness and pain for a day or two after the procedure. This procedure is sometimes combined with a *hysteroscopy*, which involves the insertion of a small telescope through the cervix into the uterine cavity so that the inside of the uterus can be seen. The diagnostic part of this procedure usually only takes about thirty minutes.

Medical Treatments

Depending on the outcome of these investigations your physician will recommend specific treatments for you or your partner. Please remember that this section is only meant to be an overview of the available treatment options. Each couple's medical situation is unique, and your health-care provider will tailor his or her recommendations to best address your specific needs and circumstances. You can learn more about the treatment options being recommended by your physician from the books in the Resources list.

If you are a man, your physician may suggest certain lifestyle changes, such as a reduction in smoking and the use of alcohol and recreational drugs, wearing boxer shorts, and staying out of hot tubs and saunas, or he or she may prescribe a round of antibiotics if there is any evidence of infection. Depending on the result of your sperm analysis *intrauterine insemination* (IUI) may be recommended. In this relatively simple procedure in the laboratory, the sperm are cleaned of any debris, concentrated, and placed directly into the woman's uterus at the time of ovulation. This may be combined with a process known as *superovulation* in which your partner is treated with medication to increase the number of eggs released in that cycle.

In other cases where a male factor problem has been identified the physician may recommend one of the advanced reproductive technologies such as *in vitro fertilization* (IVF) with *intracytoplasmic sperm injection* (ICSI). These procedures are discussed in some detail below.

If you are a woman who is not ovulating, you may be prescribed clomiphene citrate (Clomid or Serophene), a nonsteroidal, nonhormonal medication approved for induction of ovulation in women who are not ovulating but have normal estrogen levels. Although many women have no negative reactions to this medication, some report side effects such as moodiness, headaches, blurred vision, flashes of light in front of their eyes, hot flashes, abdominal bloating and discomfort, and breast tenderness. Weight gain and sleep disturbance are less commonly reported side effects of this medication. Clomiphene increases the risk of multiple births by approximately 5 to 8 percent (Corson 1999).

Approximately 70 to 80 percent of non-ovulatory women ovulate while using clomiphene citrate. However, if after taking six cycles of clomiphene you were still not ovulating, your physician would need to conduct further evaluation to identify any other contributing factors, or change the treatment strategy (Corson 1999). Depending on your partner's diagnostic status, the change of strategy might include ovulation induction with injected fertility drugs known as *gonadotropins* (LH and FSH or HCG).

Gonadotropin therapy is a routine component of the assisted reproductive treatments that require the simultaneous development and release of at least one (but often multiple) oocyte (egg). Usually administered by daily injection (because there is no oral form) during the early part of the menstrual cycle, ovulation induction therapy is associated with a number of side effects. These include exaggerated physical and psychological menstrual cycle symptoms such as breast tenderness, bloating, weight gain, and mood swings. Fortunately these symptoms are frequently less intense than those that are experienced when taking clomiphene, and in fact many women find the side effects of ovulation induction to be less bothersome than they had anticipated. However, multiple birth rates of between 20 and 30 percent are associated with this treatment (ESHRE 1999; Gleicher, Oleske, Tur-Kaspa, Vidali, and Karande 2000).

If your physician finds damage to your tubes or uterus, or you are diagnosed with *endometriosis* (a condition where the endometrial tissue that would normally line the uterus is found growing outside the uterine cavity), a recommendation may be made for surgery or drug therapy. This recommendation will depend on a number of factors including the extent of the damage, the degree of endometriosis, your age, and whether your partner has also been diagnosed with a fertility problem. IVF is the recommended treatment of choice for more severe cases of endometriosis and tubal disease (Corson 1999), with surgery often being used as a first line of treatment. If indicated, surgery to cauterize and remove the endometriosis is usually done at the time of the laparoscopy procedure.

Assisted Reproductive Technologies

A brief description of IVF and the other assisted reproductive technologies follows. If your physician recommends any of these treatments, I encourage you to refer to the works listed in the Resouces section for more detailed information on what happens during treatment and what time commitments, procedures, costs, and success rates you might expect. Many clinics also provide written information and videos to help prepare you for treatment. If you and your partner aren't certain or disagree about whether or not to proceed with the treatment your physician recommends, you might find the material in chapter 3 helpful in your decision making.

Developed in the late 1970s, IVF was originally designed as a treatment for women whose fallopian tubes were too severely blocked or damaged to be repaired by surgery. By stimulating the production of several oocytes (eggs), retrieving these oocytes from the ovaries of the woman, combining them with her partner's prepared sperm in the laboratory, and transferring the embryos to her uterus theoretically the tubal problem was bypassed.

While in vitro fertilization is still the treatment of choice in most cases of tubal disease that are not surgically correctable, and in cases of severe or extensive pelvic adhesions, IVF is also used in some cases of endometriosis, untreatable infertility, cases of ovulation failure which do not respond to other treatments, and in combination with *intracytoplasmic sperm injection* (ICSI) for the treatment of male factor problems (Corson 1999). ICSI has revolutionized the treatment of severe male factor fertility problems and is widely used in cases where a male factor has been diagnosed as the major cause of the fertility problem regardless of whether a female factor has also been identified.

In Vitro Fertilization (IVF)

An IVF cycle involves the use of naturally occurring hormones to stimulate the growth of several eggs (as opposed to the usual one egg per cycle). At the appropriate time the eggs are removed and fertilized outside of the body, and embryos are replaced into the woman's uterus. Treatment usually begins with the woman taking a drug known as a *GnRH agonist* "to shut down communications between the pituitary and the ovaries" (Corson 1999, 239). This prevents ovulation, or the release of eggs from the ovaries, from occurring during treatment before the eggs can be removed. Multiple egg growth is then stimulated using hormones known as gonadotropins, just as it is in ovulation induction, discussed earlier in the chapter under "Medical Treatments." Unlike ovulation induction, however, in IVF the goal of stimulation is to produce and retrieve more eggs since not all eggs will generally fertilize and divide in a normal fashion (Corson 1999).

People sometimes wonder why this type of medicated stimulation is necessary, and why an egg from a woman's normal cycle isn't sufficient. The reason is that usually only one egg is released in each normal cycle. Given the costs involved in retrieving, fertilizing, and replacing the embryo, and the fact that the odds of successful fertilization and implantation are significantly less with only one egg, the stimulation of several eggs provides couples with their greatest chance of success using IVF.

Once it is determined through ultrasound that the eggs are mature, a determination based on their size, they are retrieved. This involves a short procedure (fifteen to thirty minutes long) during which a physician, guided by an ultrasound image, aspirates fluid containing mature eggs from the follicles in the ovaries (spaces in which the eggs grow). Because the ovaries can be a bit sensitive and most women are understandably anxious about the procedure, most clinics administer a mild sedative and local anesthesia in order to make the process more comfortable. Some clinics also encourage women to bring in a compact disc or tape player with soothing music, to help decrease anxiety during the egg retrieval process. If you find yourself feeling anxious about the retrieval, I'd also recommend using the relaxation exercises described in chapter 4.

Unlike what can be done with unfertilized sperm and with embryos, researchers have not yet found a reliable way to freeze and thaw eggs. Consequently, at this point in the process they must be fertilized. Once the eggs are retrieved, the male partner is asked to provide a fresh semen sample. After the sample is prepared in the laboratory to recover the most motile sperm, fifty thousand to one hundred thousand sperm are placed in a laboratory dish (referred to as a Petri dish) together with each egg. Over the next twenty-four hours fertilization takes place and the eggs begin dividing to form embryos. Depending on the man's sperm parameters, the quality of the oocytes, and the age of the woman, approximately 70 to 80 percent can be expected to fertilize (Seibel 1996).

On the second or third day, following the retrieval or in some cases the fifth or sixth day (the blastocyst stage), the embryos are transferred into the woman's uterus using a catheter inserted through her cervix. Progesterone is usually given from the time of retrieval to help make the lining of the uterus more receptive to attachment. Waiting to transfer until the blastocyst stage may result in better success rates for the transferred embryos to implant, but frequently the number of embryos available for transfer is significantly decreased because a larger percentage do not develop to this stage (Corson 1999). In some cases no embryos develop to the blastocyst stage and thus no embryos are available to transfer.

It takes approximately four to six days for the embryos to implant in the wall of the uterus, and another several days before a period occurs (if no pregnancy results) or before a blood test can reveal a possible pregnancy (Corson 1999). This period is usually stressful for couples because there is little that they can do but wait to determine whether treatment has been successful. As is discussed in chapter 4, you would be well advised to maintain as normal a routine as possible during this time, maintaining a reasonable level of activity according to your physician's suggestions.

When there are embryos left over at the time of the transfer, many couples decide to have them frozen. This procedure is known as *cryopreservation.* Rates of pregnancy with previously frozen embryos are usually not as high as with fresh embryos, and some embryos do not survive the freezing and thawing process. However, many couples like to have the option of trying again with the thawed embryos. They may use the thawed embryos later if the initial IVF treatment isn't successful, or if in the future they decide to try to increase their family size after a successful IVF cycle.

The issue of what happens to frozen embryos, if couples no longer wish to use them, if they divorce, or if one partner dies, is complex. In some states this decision may be guided by legal statutes. There are also moral, ethical, and religious concerns related to the disposition of frozen embryos. If you are successful in your attempts to have a family, especially if you have twins or triplets, you may wish to donate your remaining embryos to another infertile couple. Or you may elect to donate the extra embryos for medical research. Or you may wish to have them destroyed.

Most clinics have couples sign consent forms regarding the disposition of their embryos, and many provide guidelines that are based on state laws. The American Society for Reproductive Medicine has also published guidelines regarding the disposition and use of frozen embryos (see Resources). If you and your partner are considering the option of cryopreservation you should familiarize yourselves with the laws in your state and the policies of the clinic performing this service. You should discuss your feelings regarding the use of embryos in the unlikely event that something happens to one or both of you or in the event of a divorce. Consider drawing up a notarized contract or making an amendment to your wills in order to ensure that your respective desires are documented. If you are uncertain about your options, many clinics have counselors available or can recommend counselors, with whom you can discuss these issues.

Intracytoplasmic Sperm Injection (ICSI)

This procedure is a variation of IVF and is the treatment of choice for male factor infertility and in cases where sperm must be retrieved from the testicles or the epididymis. In testicular sperm extraction (TESE), sperm are extracted from the man's testicles generally while he is under a local anesthetic. In the other two methods of sperm extraction, micro-epididymal sperm aspiration (MESA) and pecutaneous sperm aspiration (PESA) semen is aspirated from the epididymal ducts while the man is under a general or local anesthetic.

Once the sperm has been obtained, virtually the same protocol used for IVF is followed. The only difference is in the way the sperm and eggs are fertilized in the laboratory. One motile sperm is microinjected into each of the available mature eggs. As in IVF, the fertilization process takes place in the laboratory; a few days later, the embryos are transferred to the woman's uterus, where hopefully one or more may implant into her uterine wall and continue to form into a viable fetus.

The Society for Assisted Reproductive Technology, now called the American Society for Reproductive Medicine (1996), reports the average pregnancy rates of ICSI to be similar to those of IVF. Because rates can vary considerably due to factors unique to each case and to each clinic, it is recommended that you ask your physician about your probabilities of success at their clinic, given your particular diagnostic status. The information in chapter 3 may also help you to understand and interpret the success rates provided by the program you are attending.

Gamete Intrafallopian Transfer (GIFT)

In cases where the woman has at least one open fallopian tube and her partner has good sperm parameters, another variation of the IVF procedure may be recommended. This treatment is commonly known as *gamete intrafallopian transfer* (GIFT). Usually the protocol is the same as that used in IVF except that the collection of eggs is done using an ultrasound or laparoscopic procedure while the woman is under a general anesthetic. Also, the woman's eggs and the man's sperm are not fertilized in the laboratory. Rather, they are mixed together and then transferred into the fallopian tube, the place in the woman's body where conception would normally occur. Theoretically, this treatment comes closer than IVF to mimicking nature.

A major drawback of using GIFT is that it does not allow for the diagnosis of fertilization problems. Because the gametes (sperm and eggs) are placed in the woman's fallopian tube before they have fertilized, and because fertilization does not guarantee implantation, it is not possible with this procedure to determine whether or not fertilization actually occurred, in cases that don't result in a pregnancy.

Zygote Intrafallopian Transfer (ZIFT)

In another variation of the IVF procedure, zygote intrafallopian transfer (ZIFT), embryos that have been fertilized in the laboratory are placed directly into the woman's tubes, rather than into her uterus, usually using a laparoscopic procedure. The benefit of ZIFT is that fertilization problems can be identified. A major drawback is the added complexity, costs, and discomfort of the laparoscopic procedure and the need for a general anesthetic. Because reported success rates are generally no higher than those of standard IVF (Seibel 1996), ZIFT is not a commonly performed treatment.

Assisted Hatching

Another micromanipulation technique, which is becoming more common, is called *assisted embryo hatching*. When couples have been unsuccessful in achieving a pregnancy through IVF or ICSI despite having high-quality embryos, an implantation problem may be implicated. In order for implantation to occur, the embryo must break out of an outer layer known as the zona. Specialists believe that in some cases this outer layer may be too thick for the embryo to break through, thereby preventing implantation (Keye 1999). In assisted embryo hatching, specialists assist the embryos to get out of the zona, by creating a break in the zona before transferring the fertilized egg(s) into the woman's uterus. This is a relatively new technique that appears to be promising, although how significantly it can improve pregnancy rates remains to be determined.

Important Considerations

Issues to be considered with any of these assisted reproductive technologies include the cost of treatment, the possibility of multiple births, and the health of the children created through the use of these procedures. The costs of these treatments are characteristically quite high and there is no national insurance coverage in the United States or Canada for assisted reproductive technology procedures. In the United States only a handful of states (including Arkansas, Connecticut, Hawaii, Illinois, Maryland, Massachusetts, Rhode Island, and Texas) have introduced bills requiring insurance companies to provide coverage for some of these procedures. In Canada, public health care coverage for assisted reproductive technologies is available only in the province of Ontario for women with both tubes blocked, although some extended health-care plans cover part of the costs of the required medications and some of the procedures (e.g., ultrasound testing).

Some American fertility centers offer to defer some or all of the costs of a treatment cycle if couples are willing to donate a percentage of their oocytes (eggs) to another couple. In exchange for this donation the recipient couple pays the cost of their own treatment cycle as well as the cycle of the donor. The ethical and moral issues involved in this type of arrangement have been widely debated in the field of reproductive medicine and are understandably quite complex (Andereck, Thomasma, Goldworth, and Kushner, 1998). Couples who are considering this option are usually asked to meet with a counselor to address these issues prior to proceeding with treatment.

With the assistance of these reproductive technologies comes an increased chance of having multiple fetuses. After years of trying to have a baby, a couple can find it difficult to decide between selectively reducing a multiple-fetus pregnancy and maintaining a multiple pregnancy, with all the attendant risks (the possibility of miscarriage in the first trimester, or giving birth to sick or very premature babies). Limiting the number of embryos transferred to the uterus reduces the likelihood of being faced with this difficult dilemma.

Concerns have also been raised about the health of babies conceived with the assistance of these technologies. In particular, the process in which single sperm are selected in a laboratory and used in the fertilization process, rather than the sperm making its own way to the egg as it would in a natural conception, have raised questions about whether we are interfering with the process of natural selection. Fortunately, data gathered over the last decade seem to suggest that children conceived through IVF and ICSI have no greater risk of birth defects than do children conceived through intercourse (Keye 1999).

Third-Party Reproductive Options

Depending on your diagnosis, you may be faced with the decision to use the contribution of a third person to help create your family. These are usually referred to as third-party reproductive options because they involve the use of donor sperm, donor eggs, donor embryos, a gestational carrier, a surrogate, or some combination of these options. None of these options are easy to embrace at first, but for many couples they provide hope and opportunity for creating a family.

Most couples are not comfortable pursuing these alternatives until they feel they have done everything possible to try to produce a child who would share their genetic histories. If you are faced with having to use any of the options discussed below to help you create your family, avoid rushing right into treatment. Before proceeding with any of these options, be sure both you and your partner are comfortable with your decision, and that you have had an opportunity to consider the range of issues, feelings, and concerns regarding the short- and long-term consequences of your treatment choice. It pays in the long run to take some time to deal with the wide range of feelings and fears you both will likely have about this choice. Give yourselves time to work through these feelings and deal with your loss of the possibility of having a child who is biologically related to both of you, so that if you do go ahead with treatment, you can both delight in becoming parents together when you finally learn that you are pregnant. The case of Ted and Susan is a good example of what can happen when couples rush too quickly into a treatment option they're not emotionally prepared for.

After Ted, thirty-six, was diagnosed as having a very low sperm count, he and his wife Susan, twenty-nine, pursued several rounds of intrauterine insemination using Ted's sperm. When this wasn't successful they decided to try one cycle of IVF using ICSI. Although they were aware that the odds of success were only about 35 to 40 percent, they felt they needed to try this treatment once, for closure. When it didn't work, at Ted's insistence they immediately began treatment using donor sperm. When Susan became pregnant in the second cycle of treatment, Ted was overwhelmed with feelings of inadequacy. After five years of trying to have a child, he was emotionally unprepared for his feelings when Susan so easily became pregnant using donor sperm. Susan was delighted to finally be pregnant, but she was frightened by Ted's negative reaction to their pregnancy. During counseling, Ted and Susan both had to work through their feelings of grief at being unable to produce a child who shared their genetic histories, and Ted had to seriously consider how important genetic ties were in his desire for, and understanding of fatherhood, a subject that is addressed in chapter 3. Only then were they both able to accept and delight in their pregnancy.

Donor Sperm

From a technical standpoint, using donor sperm is considered one of the easiest, least invasive, and most successful ways for couples with an obvious male factor fertility problem, or couples in which the man may carry a lethal or severe genetic abnormality, to conceive a child. Emotionally, however, it is usually a very difficult choice for couples. The emotional and social issues related to the use of the sperm of a known or unknown donor are discussed in chapter 3. The medical pragmatics of using donor sperm are addressed below.

People are often surprised to learn that the option of using donor sperm has been available in North America since the early 1960s. Typically, this was accomplished through the anonymous donations of medical students. More recently, however, a number of large commercial sperm banks have been established. These banks use the sperm collected from donors who have been screened for a wide range of genetic diseases, infections, and health problems.

Until the mid-1980s fresh sperm was usually used. However, because of the outbreak of AIDS and our knowledge of other sexually transmitted diseases such as chlamydia and hepatitis B and C, the use of fresh sperm has been prohibited in some parts of the world (e.g., Canada). It also contravenes the guidelines for therapeutic donor insemination of the American Society for Reproductive Medicine (1998), which recommend that sperm be quarantined for at least six months and donors be tested at the time of sperm donation, and then retested for HIV and other sexually transmitted diseases six months later, prior to the frozen sperm being released for use by the recipient. Some loss in sperm motility and efficiency occurs as a consequence of freezing; however, with millions of available sperm in each sample, this doesn't appear to significantly affect success rates.

When a commercial bank is used, you can select a donor after reading a number of profiles describing the donor's physical characteristics, family health history, education, occupation, interests, etc. Depending on the bank, more or less information may be available on each donor. In some centers, however, anonymous local donors are used and you are given little or no choice in the selection of the donor, and no information about the donor's genetic or health background.

Many couples considering the use of donor sperm are concerned about the number of recipients who are allowed to use the same donor. Fortunately, many programs limit the number of families each donor can contribute to, in an effort to reduce the likelihood that children conceived using the same donor might inadvertently end up partnering with each other when they become adults.

Many people also wonder why men elect to be sperm donors. Certainly donors are usually compensated financially for their time and expenses, but this compensation tends to be quite minimal (e.g., $40 to $75 per donation). As a consequence, most men who contribute to donor programs do so because they are aware of the pain and disappointment felt by friends or family members who are unable to have children. Some enjoy being parents themselves and want to help other people to experience pregnancy and parenthood.

The price of treatment using donor sperm usually includes the cost of the sperm, monitoring of ovulation, and the cost of the insemination. Some fertility centers also require that you participate in an orientation visit and counseling session prior to undertaking this treatment. This session can be a good opportunity to discuss any questions or concerns you have regarding donor selection and regarding the issue of whether and how much you elect to tell the child and significant others in your life about the child's genetic origin.

Once a donor has been selected, ovulation is monitored by urine or blood testing. When ovulation is detected, the sperm is thawed and placed either into the woman's vagina and held in place by a cervical cup or, more commonly, directly into the uterus with the assistance of a small catheter. For women under forty years of age, per-cycle success rates using the intrauterine approach are between 10 and 20 percent. A successful pregnancy is usually achieved within six cycles of treatment in 50 to 60 percent of women.

Donor Eggs

In cases where egg development cannot be stimulated (e.g., premature ovarian failure or menopause), or the quality of eggs being produced is not satisfactory, the use of donor eggs may be an option. If a severe male factor problem has also been identified the use of donor eggs can sometimes be combined with ICSI. In some instances both donor eggs and donor sperm may be required where there are egg and sperm problems.

As with donor sperm, the social and emotional issues surrounding this form of treatment are complex. Issues you need to consider are addressed in chapter 3. This option is also considerably more complex from a medical standpoint than the use of donor sperm because it requires the egg donor to be stimulated with the same hormone medications used in a standard IVF cycle. The donor must also go through the egg-retrieval process. As the recipient, you would also be treated with hormone medications to control your pituitary functioning and to prepare your uterine lining for a possible pregnancy. The eggs retrieved from the donor would then be combined with your partner's sperm (or donor sperm), and some of the resulting fertilized embryos would be transferred to your uterus. You could choose to freeze the remainder for use at a later date.

Egg donors may be known or anonymous. Given the invasiveness of this form of treatment, it is not uncommon for a known donor to be a close friend or a family member (often a sister). Many centers also offer the option of using the eggs of an unknown donor. The degree of choice and the amount of information available to you for selecting a donor varies considerably among facilities. Ideally, the donor will be under thirty-five years of age and have proven fertility (a previous viable pregnancy).

Egg donation has only recently become more widely available. Guidelines have been established by the American Society for Reproductive Medicine (1998) for the selection, screening, and compensation of egg donors. These guidelines recommend genetic and psychological screening. However, the degree to which these guidelines are followed may vary among clinics, so it is advisable to inquire about the screening and assessment of donors if you are considering this option.

Average success rates of egg donation programs are similar to or higher than those for standard IVF. Recently some clinics have reported success rates for oocyte donor cycles in excess of 60 percent. However, success rates tend to be quite dependent on the age and fertility status of the donors. In cases where the donor is under thirty-five years of age, has previously given birth to a healthy child or children, and has no family history of premature ovarian failure, success rates tend to be higher (sometimes as high as 35 to 40 percent). For donors over thirty-five, the rates are often lower (Seibel 1996).

The issue of cost is also complex. Most programs will charge you, the recipient couple, for all of the fees related to the treatment cycle, including donor screening, hormones, ovulation monitoring, egg recovery, embryo transfer, and all laboratory work. Additionally, if the donor is anonymous you will be expected or required to compensate the donor for her direct and indirect expenses including her inconvenience, time, physical discomfort, and additional medical and counseling expenses. Payment is usually required, even if no eggs are retrieved and the cycle has to be canceled.

Donor Embryos

A very recent development is the use of embryos donated by other couples who no longer wish to use the cryopreserved embryos left over from their previous IVF treatment cycles. Currently, for a range of ethical, moral, and religious reasons, few couples are willing to donate their embryos.

The American Society for Reproductive Medicine (1998) published guidelines for embryo donation that cover the acceptable criteria for the program handling the embryo donation, for the couple donating their embryos, and for the recipient couple. The few clinics that offer this option each have their own protocols and may elect to restrict access to couples of a certain age or marital status.

According to the ASRM guidelines for embryo donation (1998), embryos need to have been cryopreserved for at least two and not more than five years. At the time the embryos were created, the woman of the donor couple should have been less than forty years old. The donors usually submit to a number of tests for infectious diseases, blood typing, and HIV. They also undergo counseling, and they sign a consent form relinquishing all rights to the embryos and to any child or children produced with their embryos. Similar to organ donation, embryo donation is considered a gift in kind. As such, donors usually are not compensated.

If you use donated embryos you may have some limited opportunity to match your traits and characteristics and those of your partner with those of the donor couple (e.g., race, ethnicity, physical characteristics, and so on). Once the donor couple has been selected, you essentially go through the same procedures you would if you were using your own cryopreserved embryos.

The cost of this process varies from clinic to clinic. However, because of the limited amount of direct intervention and medications required, it is usually less expensive than a standard cycle of IVF. However, numerous complex issues may arise for you and your partner, and for the child(ren) you create using donated embryos. Consequently, most programs have counselors who can help you and your partner work through these issues when you are considering donating embryos, or using donated embryos.

Gestational Carrier

If you do not have a uterus or your uterus can't carry a pregnancy, the only option available, if you want to have a genetically related child, is to use a gestational carrier. This requires that you have at least one functioning ovary.

First you would go through the initial stages of IVF to the point of egg retrieval and fertilization with your partner's sperm. Your embryos would then be transferred to the uterus of the gestational carrier, a woman whose uterus has been prepared with hormones in order to synchronize her cycle with yours and make her uterus more receptive to a pregnancy. She then carries the pregnancy to term and turns the child over to you and your partner when the baby is born, relinquishing all legal rights to the child.

One of the difficulties of this form of treatment is finding a woman who is willing to carry a pregnancy and relinquish the child at birth. Some clinics help couples find willing carriers, while others insist that couples find their own carrier. Considerable legal and emotional issues are involved, since the child is genetically related to you, rather than to the woman who carries and gives birth to the child. Getting legal assistance with the contractual arrangements is critical. Counseling is also highly recommended in all cases. It is also important to note that gestational care arrangements are not legal in some states.

The costs for this form of treatment tend to be quite high. They include the expenses for IVF as well as compensation to the carrier for her role in carrying the child, and all of the medical costs related to the delivery. These costs usually apply, irrespective of the health of the child or children born.

Surrogacy

Surrogacy is another parenting option if you are diagnosed with an irreparable problem to your uterus and ovaries. A woman who is known or hired by you and your partner is inseminated with your partner's sperm. The surrogate carries the child, who is half genetically related to her and half related to your partner. When the baby is born, she turns the child over to you and relinquishes all legal rights to the child.

Medically, this is a much easier and less invasive procedure than those that require the use of assisted reproductive technology. However, because of your child's genetic relationship to the surrogate, and the surrogate's emotional relationship to the child, this process is associated with many social, legal, and ethical issues. It can also be very costly, because of the compensation paid to the surrogate. If you are considering surrogacy I'd strongly advise you to seek legal advice and psychological support for yourselves and for your surrogate. More detailed information on this option can be found in the Resource section.

Conclusion

It can be helpful to know what decisions and treatments might be in store following the medical evaluation of your fertility problems. It can also be reassuring to know that a number of treatment options exist to assist you in your efforts to create your family. However, coping with the stresses of infertility and medical testing, and making informed and satisfying decisions regarding the available treatment options are not always easy. The information in the following chapters is provided to assist you in your decision making and to help you cope with the stresses of medical testing and treatments.

3

Making Decisions You Can Live With

When you begin fertility investigations and treatments you will be faced with decisions you could never have imagined when you first began this process. After all, whether you always knew you wanted children or not, the decision to change your lives and start a family is challenging enough. Do we want kids? How many do we want? Is now the right time? Is one of us going to stay home with the kids? Which one? For how long? The choices aren't easy at the best of times, but when you enter the world of medical fertility treatment, they become even more difficult. How badly do we want to be parents? Should we take this test? What do the results mean? Should we try this treatment? How many times? What about side effects? What are our chances of success? Is it right to be doing this? Is it ethical? Can we afford to do this? Can we afford not to do this? How badly do we want to be parents? How important is it that the child be genetically related to one or both of us? Could we love a child who isn't our own? Will we regret it if we don't try everything? How badly do we want to be parents?

These questions are bewildering, and there are no easy answers. The assisted reproductive technologies are relatively recent, so it is hard to base your decisions on the experiences of others who have walked in your shoes. New tests are developed and treatment options are refined each year. In some ways you're like pioneers, facing decisions that few people have had to face, often without a lot of information on the long-term consequences of your choices.

The issue of choice related to your infertility can be somewhat of a double-edged sword. On the one hand, it is a relief to know that medical science keeps forging ahead and coming up with new diagnostic procedures and treatments to combat infertility. On the other hand, this very fact can make it extremely difficult to decide which treatments you're willing to pursue, and when to stop and move on.

Making decisions about fertility treatments and parenting options is best viewed as a process that evolves over time. It is a process that changes you and your partner, and it forces you to confront your basic beliefs and values—about yourselves and what it means to be a parent. You want to make the right decisions, both for emotional and financial reasons. Most important, you want to make decisions that you both can live with—without regrets. The suggestions in this chapter are meant to guide you in this process.

"We Never Thought We'd Be Doing This": Keeping Your Options Open

When I talk with couples who are at the beginning of their medical investigation they are usually quite optimistic that answers will be found explaining why they aren't getting pregnant. Most have heard stories about the amazing advancements scientists have made in the area of reproductive technology, and they have faith that, once the problem is diagnosed, medicine will have a solution to their problem. They expect that the process of identifying their problem and finding solutions will be relatively short, and that within a year they'll likely be pregnant.

They also usually have clear ideas of how far they're willing to go in their efforts to produce a child—many saying that they'd never consider using the more advanced technologies such as in vitro fertilization (IVF), and certainly not third-party reproductive options like donor eggs or sperm. Many are surprised to find themselves, several months or years later, considering treatment and parenting options that, at the beginning, they were absolutely certain they'd never consider. Rod, a forty-two-year-old carpenter, reflects on his surprise to find himself considering the use of donor sperm:

> You know, if somebody had told me that we'd ever consider donor sperm I'd have said they were crazy. We wanted a child that was our child—one with our characteristics—the good and the bad! We didn't want some stranger's genes. We even talked about it at the beginning and said, okay, we'll try ICSI,

but only once. And then before we knew it, we'd done it three times, and we still didn't have a baby. We were devastated. So we took some time to consider our options, and here we are a year later, ready to do donor sperm. Who would have believed it?

To your surprise you and your partner may find yourselves accepting your situation and reassessing your priorities regarding parenthood as you work your way through the "minefield" of medical testing and treatment. Coping with infertility and dealing with the many losses associated with not being able to produce a child "naturally" is something that takes time. Accepting the reality of your infertility, and making decisions about how important children are in your lives, and how far you're willing to go in your efforts to become parents, is a complicated process that seems even more difficult because the outcome isn't certain. The decisions you will face down the road depend on the choices you make now, and how these turn out. So, you can't really know what choices you'll make later until you've lived through and know the consequences of your current choices. It's a series of decisions that you have to make, one by one, based on what you'd hoped for, what you've already tried, and what your options are next. Here's how the series of decisions frequently plays out:

First, you have to deal with the fact that without medical assistance you may never be able to have children. If conception happens at all, it will likely occur in a physician's office or a laboratory! So much for romantic notions of unbridled passion, or planning the birth of your child for when it would best fit into your lives. You have no desire to medicalize such an intimate and important event as the conception of your child, but you come to realize that if you're going to have any chance of having a baby, you're just going to have to deal with the indignities of having the most private aspects of your bodies and lives together subjected to medical scrutiny. So you book an appointment with a fertility specialist and begin the process of searching for answers and solutions.

You and your partner are intimidated by or concerned about some of the diagnostic tests, like the hysterosalpingogram (HSG) or the testicular biopsy, but you also realize that without these tests, your physician won't be able to explain why you're not getting pregnant, much less suggest how to fix the problem. So you find yourselves going through a battery of tests. You are opposed to taking fertility drugs, concerned about the short- and long-term effects of these medications, but find yourself taking clomiphene pills or injecting yourself with fertility medications. You also aren't keen on using high-tech interventions, believing that it isn't right or natural to be interfering with nature, yet find yourself planning an IVF treatment cycle. The words of Mary, a thirty-three-year-old lawyer, capture the reality of the struggle:

> I was really leery of Pergonal because I had done a bit of research and didn't really like what my body was going to be invaded by and what it was going to be forced to do. And I worried about what might happen down to the road—to me, and to the child if we were lucky enough to get pregnant. I mean, after all, how do we know that this stuff doesn't affect the fetus? So we talked it over and weighed the risks, but we went ahead with IVF. I was scared, but the drive to have a child was stronger than my fear of the drugs.

You attempt to assess the information and recommendations made by your fertility specialist, and you try to make informed decisions. You carefully consider your options—treatment versus potential childlessness. You weigh the success rates, hoping that, if the chance of success is one in five, you're going to be the one. Before you know it, and much to your surprise, you find yourselves undergoing a form of treatment that a year or two ago you never would have considered. Perhaps you even find yourselves considering using the sperm or eggs or uterus of someone else to help you create a child.

So, Why Do You Do It?

You do it because you believe you have a chance of success. You do it because there is a chance of success. You do it because you want to be parents. You do it because, when all is said and done, you don't want to look back in a few years and wonder, "What if we'd tried it? What if it had worked?" If it doesn't work the first time you may even do it again, because this time you feel you might be the lucky ones—this time it might be your turn. You do it because, after investing so much time and money in pursuing solutions to your infertility, it's hard to walk away now.

You do it because you're terrified of having to face the fact that you might never have your own biological children—never know what it's like to feel or watch a child grow inside you, or your partner, never go through childbirth together, never see the things you love about your partner, or the generations that came before you, reflected in your child. You do it because to not do it means letting go of a dream and facing an uncertain future, one that may never include children.

Be prepared to take this one step at a time—one decision at a time. You can't possibly know now what you and your partner will be willing to consider later. You also can't know how you're going to feel about a particular option until you've worked your way through the other steps in the process. When you're at a stage in the process where you believe you'll never have to face a choice like high-tech treatment, or selective reduction, it is easy to dismiss such a treatment. However, when it becomes your only choice for starting a family, or saving a pregnancy, or having a healthy child, dismissing it is not so easy.

Another important reason to take this one step at a time is that the decisions being made are joint decisions made by you and your partner, based on both of your needs and experiences. When you prematurely close the door on a future treatment or parenting option, later on it can be much harder to agree on the next step, especially when one of you is ready to reconsider a previously discarded option, but the other is not.

Understanding Your Decision-Making Styles

Every person and every couple facing infertility is different. Each has a different way of coping with the experience, a different way of making decisions. There is no right or wrong way to decide these issues. It is important to be aware of your own personal decision making style, as well as that of your partner. For example, one of you may find that you need to have more than one option available to you in case your most desired option isn't successful. Your particular style of coping with the stress and uncertainty may be to have a "plan B" in place, so that if your current treatment option isn't successful, you know that there is still another course of action to take. Or you may be the type of person who copes best by dealing with the decision at hand, rather than allowing yourself to be distracted by the choices that you might have to face in the future.

Applying for adoption while still pursuing fertility treatment is an example of how different decision-making styles can affect the choices you make. While you are going through fertility investigations and treatments you may feel a need to start the adoption process, even before you have exhausted all your treatment options or have learned whether treatment will be successful. Applying for adoption while still pursuing treatment may serve to reassure you that, one way or the other, your dreams of being parents together will be realized.

On the other hand, you may not be able to even consider this option while you're still pursuing treatment. You and your partner may not be ready to give up your dream of having a baby together, and you may feel that applying for adoption before you've done everything possible to produce your own biological child would be like giving up. Or perhaps you both feel that treatment is taking up so much space in your lives that you just don't have the emotional energy to pursue another parenting option. Maybe you cope best when you have only one option to think about at a time. You may feel you need all of your energy to be sure you're giving this treatment your very best effort, and that you'll consider other parenting options only if all of the medical treatments fail.

Another example is the decision to have donor sperm as a backup option when you are going through IVF and ICSI and there is a possibility that there won't be enough live sperm available to fertilize the eggs that are retrieved. Even though you haven't abandoned the idea of having your own child together, you and your partner may decide that using donor sperm would be your next choice if ICSI isn't successful. Given the financial and emotional costs of an IVF/ICSI cycle, you may be willing to select a donor to be used as a backup, so that the eggs that are retrieved are not "wasted."

On the other hand, you and your partner may not be emotionally ready to take this step. You may not be comfortable with having donor sperm as a backup option, even if there is a good chance that not enough viable sperm will be available to fertilize the eggs. You may be committed to doing all you can to produce your own genetic offspring first, needing to do this first before you will be ready to consider other parenting options.

Every couple is different. There is no one right way to make decisions or to approach infertility. People come into this with different decision making and coping styles—different styles that work for them. So rather than compare yourselves to other couples, it is important to know what works best for you and your partner.

One good way to do this is to look back at other important decisions you've made in your life. How did you select your line of work? How did you decide to end a relationship that wasn't working for you? How did you make the decision to move to a different city, buy your car, or make a commitment to your partner? Are you the type of person who labors over decisions, weighing the pros and cons, perhaps writing them down on a piece of paper? Or are you the type who makes quick, spontaneous decisions using your intuition? Are you a risk taker, or do you tend to play it safe when it comes to making important life decisions? Overall, have you been pretty satisfied with your choices? If so, then obviously your style of decision making has worked for you in the past, and it will likely serve you well in this situation.

What about your partner? How does he or she make important life decisions? Are your styles similar or different? As a couple, how have you made critical decisions in the past, especially those that you're both satisfied with? Answering these questions can help you to predict how you'll make satisfying decisions about your fertility and parenting options.

Information Is Power: Getting the Information You Need

When it comes to making decisions about fertility treatments, it is important to be an informed consumer. Most fertility specialists are very busy, and try as you might, getting all your questions answered can be difficult. If you are going to make informed treatment decisions, it is important to do three things:

1. Make a list of the questions you need answered and bring it with you to your medical consultations. Writing down your questions about your particular situation, diagnosis, or treatment options in advance will help to ensure that you get the answers you need. Try to prioritize your questions, because your physician may not have time to answer all of your questions during one visit.

2. Don't attend your medical consultations alone. This is especially critical when you are receiving diagnostic information or discussing the available treatment options. Be sure to attend the consultation with your partner or, if your partner is unable to attend, with a trusted friend or family member. A companion can provide valuable emotional support should you hear news you weren't expecting or were hoping not to hear. This person can also serve as a second pair of ears, as well as offering a second perspective on the information that was provided during the consultation. When faced with a

medical or personal crisis, many people will forget some of what they are told during a medical consultation, especially if they are distressed by the news they're receiving. Having someone to compare recollections with, and even asking that person to take notes during the appointment, can help ensure that the information you recall is accurate and that you remember all the information you need in order to make informed treatment choices.

3. Educate yourselves about the recommended treatments, the potential risks and side effects, and the probability of a successful pregnancy given your specific situation (e.g., age, diagnostic status, or fertility history). Don't rely on the medical staff to provide all the information you need to make an informed decision, and don't base your decisions on concerns that you'd be letting your doctor down by deciding against a particular option. If you do, and treatment doesn't work or you experience consequences you weren't expecting, you'll probably feel angry and manipulated. Ask the clinic or physician you're working with for any pamphlets or brochures they have about the recommended procedures, tests, and treatments. Be sure your partner also reads this information, or, when you have your partner's undivided attention for a few minutes, read it to him or her. Also, make a point of reading some of the recent books that describe not just the *medical*, but also the *social* and *emotional* aspects of the treatments you're considering (see Resources).

"What Are Our Chances?": Learning to Interpret Success Rates

Whether or not you believe a treatment has a chance of being successful, and whether you assess that chance as being *good enough*, are often based on feelings—faith, hope, desire, fear, and sometimes desperation. These decisions are also based on your perceptions of the odds of success for the treatment in general, and for the clinic in particular.

Making a decision like this might seem fairly straightforward, a matter of asking how often does this treatment work and for whom? But in fact, interpreting success rates is not so easy. Let's use IVF as an example. Clinics frequently report their success rates using the average number of pregnancies they have achieved per IVF treatment cycle performed—the pregnancy rate—rather than the average number of births they have achieved per treatment cycle—the live birth rate. Because approximately 20 percent of pregnancies end in miscarriage during the first three months (sometimes referred to as clinical pregnancies), the live-birth rate is always lower than the pregnancy rate. This is an important distinction. The differences between per-cycle pregnancy rates and live-birth rates, or "take-home baby rates" as they are sometimes called, can be significant.

Success rates also differ because of the woman's age. Women over forty had an average live-birth rate of 6.7 percent in 1993 for each treatment cycle. Despite advancements in technology, these rates did not increase significantly between 1993 and 2000. And as women age, the incidence of miscarriage increases substantially, especially in women over forty. For women of forty-two or older, the miscarriage rate is over 50 percent (Seibel 1996). If clinics report their pregnancy rates rather than live-birth rates, then the pregnancy rates for women over forty will be significantly higher than the actual live birth rates.

The situation can be even more confusing because the success rates quoted by clinics may be based on the number of patients who have undergone treatment, the number of eggs retrieved, or the number of embryos transferred. Dr. Machelle Seibel (1988) helps to explain the differences:

> Let's pretend a new IVF clinic has one patient who goes through the procedure five times. The first time, they fail to retrieve an egg, and the second time, the retrieved eggs fail to fertilize. The last three cycles result in embryo transfers and the patient conceives on her fifth attempt. What is the success rate? . . . The IVF success rate is one pregnancy per five oocyte retrievals or 20 percent, one pregnancy per three embryo transfers or 33 percent, or one pregnancy per one patient or 100 percent. (2)

Success rates can mean very different things, depending on what procedures the clinic in question uses to calculate their figures. Clinics may or may not include in their calculations the couples who didn't achieve fertilization or those women whose treatment cycle was cancelled because of poor response to the medication. Or they may calculate their success rates using the results from a period of time (a month, a quarter, or a year) when their pregnancy or live birth rates were high.

If you are basing your decision to pursue a particular treatment on the success rates reported by the clinic you're attending, be sure you understand what these rates really mean. If you are having diffi-culty getting or interpreting this information, you might want to con-tact the American Society for Reproductive Medicine, your local chapter of RESOLVE, or, in Canada, the Infertility Awareness Associ-ation (see Resources).

"Can We Afford to Do This?": Assessing the Many Costs of Treatment

Pursuing medical solutions to your fertility problems can be a very costly venture. Many insurers do not cover the costs of fertility drugs or high-tech procedures like IVF. With per-cycle success rates often in the 20-percent range, it may take several cycles of treatment to secure a viable pregnancy. The average cost of a live birth through IVF in the United States is estimated to be close to $66,000 (Garcia 1998). Because of the high costs involved, you may find yourselves unable to afford the treatments that offer you your best chance of achieving a pregnancy.

Like many couples, you may end up going into considerable debt to finance your fertility treatments, debt that adds to the already significant stress of being unable to have a baby. While one can never put a price on the life of a child, the financial burden must be evalu-ated relative to the probability of a successful outcome, and what you can live with. For example, even if you have to go into debt, and even if the odds of success aren't great, you might decide to try IVF so that you would have peace of mind knowing that you tried everything you could. On the other hand, you might decide that the likelihood of high-tech treatment working for you just doesn't justify the costs. Even if you can afford to try IVF, you and your partner may decide to use donor sperm (in the case of a male factor problem) or pursue adoption—putting the money instead toward the costs of the adop-tion or of raising a child. Or you may decide to construct your lives without children.

As noted in chapter 2, some fertility centers will defer the costs of your treatment cycle if you agree to donate a percentage of your eggs to another patient. While this option may help relieve the finan-cial burden of treatment, it comes with weighty ethical and moral issues to be considered. Certainly you'll have to decide how much any child produced using your eggs will be permitted to know about his or her genetic background. Most clinics have counselors who can help you consider these issues before you agree to make this type of donation.

Other clinics have responded to the increasing costs of IVF, and the fact that for many couples two or three treatment cycles are necessary to secure a pregnancy, by offering shared-risk programs. These programs are also known as warranty or refund programs. At the outset of treatment you would pay a set fee, sometimes more than twice the standard per-cycle price. The clinic then performs one cycle of IVF treatment. If you achieve a pregnancy, you forfeit the entire fee. If you do not, the clinic reimburses 80 percent to 100 percent of your original payment. This type of arrangement might be acceptable to you. However, before proceeding, discuss the specifics of the reimbursement policy with the clinic staff. For example, some clinics only guarantee a pregnancy up to twelve weeks of gestation. This means if you became pregnant and then miscarried at thirteen weeks, you would still pay the entire fee. Also, many clinics do not include the costs of the medications or diagnostic tests in their shared-risk programs. This means that only a portion of your total costs would be refunded, if the treatment did not result in a pregnancy. Other hidden costs are not reimbursed, such as time away from work and travel costs. "Buyer beware" is good advice to use when you are considering these programs. For information on the clinics that provide these shared-risk and partial donation programs you can contact the American Society for Reproductive Medicine or RESOLVE (see Resources).

As well as financial costs, the substantial emotional costs of infertility treatment need to be taken into account when you are deciding whether to pursue or abandon treatment. Infertility and medical treatment will likely take up an enormous amount of space in your lives. It may be all-consuming. The words of Jackie, a thirty-nine-year-old social worker, reflect this painful reality:

> We got to the point where we had nothing else. Everything had kind of disappeared. We woke up in the morning with it. We went to bed with it at night. Every day we were talking about it. It was everything to us. And it got to be so big, so huge really, that we weren't a couple anymore. We were just two people trying to chip away at this tremendous boulder in front of us . . . and it became a terrible thing.

Months or years of having the most intimate aspects of your lives subjected to medical scrutiny, the pressure of having to have intercourse on schedule, and the continual disappointments of failed treatment take a tremendous toll on you personally, and on your relationship. In fact, the pressures are often so great that some couples don't survive it. They find that they've lost all the fun, laughter, and joy that once were a part of their lives together. Their marriages fall apart. Other couples who do survive it say that infertility is one of the most challenging things they've ever gone through together.

In making decisions about the pursuit of treatment, then, it is important at each stage of the process to take the emotional costs, and the cost to your relationship, into consideration and to weigh these against the potential costs of not pursuing the available options. Think about whether you'll be able to live with yourselves if you don't pursue the available treatment options. Although these costs aren't always easy to see or assess, they are tremendously important to examine, especially if you don't want to lose yourself or your relationship in the process.

"But Is It Right?": Assessing the Ethical and Religious Implications

It is certainly true that medical science has advanced rapidly in the diagnosis and treatment of fertility problems, providing new hope for many infertile couples. However, when you are considering the use of some of these procedures to create a family, you may well be confronted with difficult ethical, moral, or religious dilemmas. Is it right to intervene with nature? Is it ethical to create embryos in a laboratory dish or inject eggs with sperm that have been individually selected? Is it appropriate to destroy embryos when you don't want to use them anymore, to donate them to another couple, or to let them be used for research? Is it immoral to selectively reduce a triplet pregnancy to make it more viable for the other two embryos? Is sex selection ever justifiable? Is it right to use someone else's eggs, sperm, or uterus to create a child? What about the rights of the children produced through third-party reproduction? Do they have a right to know about the circumstances of their conception? Do they have a right to information about the genetic and health history of the donor? What about your rights as the parents—do you have a right to maintain privacy and not disclose this information to the child? Is it ethical to ask a woman to carry a child for you and then relinquish that child after giving birth? Does she deserve to be compensated for her efforts? In what way?

The questions are numerous and there are no easy answers. The American Society for Reproductive Medicine has attempted to address many of these issues in its published ethical guidelines and practice standards (see Resources for information on contacting the ASRM). However, you and your partner come to this with your own beliefs and values, your own religious and moral perspectives, and these must be taken into consideration when deciding upon a course of treatment you both can live with.

Ethical and moral dilemmas are often difficult to articulate. Frequently they come out as a general sense of discomfort with a particular option, without a clear sense of where that discomfort is coming from. You may not know exactly why you're uncomfortable with a particular treatment option, but you just "don't feel right about it." It usually means you need to delve a little deeper to find the source of your discomfort. It may be fear of the unknown; it may be grief over being unable to produce a child; it may be that the option in question is against your cultural or religious beliefs; or it may be that some part of the procedure doesn't seem moral or ethical. Mentally walking through the procedure step by step is often the best way to identify and articulate the real source of your discomfort. The following three stories are examples of how some clients have identified and worked through some complex dilemmas.

Charlie, a thirty-seven-year-old engineer diagnosed with a low sperm count, was very opposed to trying IVF. He couldn't say why, he was just against it. It wasn't "natural," it wasn't "right," and it wasn't for him. During counseling we explored his feelings of discomfort. Charlie had been raised as a Catholic and he knew that the Catholic Church does not support the use of IVF, but that wasn't what was bothering him. He concurred with the Catholic belief that the creation of life is holy, but he didn't believe the children produced through IVF were less worthy because of the technology used to help in their creation. Science also wasn't a problem for him. Similar to his belief about heart transplants, Charlie's philosophy about IVF was that God wouldn't have given people the skills and knowledge to develop this type of technology if He didn't want us to use it. So it wasn't the use of technology that he was opposed to. Rather, it was that Charlie believed life began at the moment of conception. He believed that embryos created in the lab constituted life and should not be destroyed. On the basis of this understanding, he and his partner came to an agreement that if they went through IVF they would limit the number of oocytes to be transferred, not reduce a multiple pregnancy, and not allow the extra embryos to be destroyed.

In another situation, forty-three-year-old Jan was really struggling with the idea of using her sister's eggs to help her have a child. As she explored this issue more deeply it became apparent that her discomfort was not based, as she initially thought, on moral or ethical issues. Rather, it had to do with her concerns about her gestational versus genetic relationship with the child, and with her sister's potential feelings about, and relationship with, the child. However, after thoroughly discussing her feelings with her partner and with her sister, she came to some peace with this option. She came to believe that by carrying the child in her body, she would indeed be passing on her blood, her thoughts, and her essence to the child. She realized that if the tables were turned, she'd gladly donate her eggs to help her sister become a mother. She found comfort in the knowledge that, although her child would not have her genes, the child would share her family's genetic history.

Greg, a twenty-nine-year-old professional athlete, had always dreamed of one day coaching his son. He hoped his natural athletic ability would be passed on to his child. It came as a tremendous shock when he was diagnosed as having no sperm (azoospermic). Adoption or the use of donor sperm were his only parenting options. His wife, Linda, twenty-seven, was keen to experience pregnancy and didn't want to deal with the scrutiny and uncertainty of the adoption process. She was willing to use donor sperm but Greg just did not feeling right about this option. As he explored his discomfort a bit further he realized that it wasn't because he couldn't love a child who was not genetically related to him. Yes, he was disappointed that his genes wouldn't be passed on, but he felt that he could still teach his son or daughter to develop a passion for sports. And a child was a child. He loved his nieces and nephews and they loved him, so he knew he could love any child, especially one produced by his wife Linda. He finally concluded that his discomfort was based on his religious beliefs that using donor sperm was against God's will. When he spoke with his minister about his concerns, he was surprised at the minister's response. The minister asked him if he believed in the soul. Greg said, "Yes, absolutely." He then asked if he believed that the body is merely the house of the soul. Again, Greg said, "Yes." The minister then said, "There is a little soul out there waiting to be a part of your life. Does it really matter whether the body that little soul inhabits is made up of your genes?"

Like the men and women in these examples, if you or your partner find that you are concerned about the ethics or morality of a particular treatment option, you need to heed this discomfort and take some time to explore the source and nature of your feelings. Sometimes just getting more specific information about the treatment can help to identify the specific nature of your struggle. In their book *Beyond Infertility: The New Paths to Parenthood* (1994) Susan Cooper and Elen Glazer do a very good job of addressing many of the more difficult and controversial aspects of using advanced reproductive technologies and the third-party reproductive options of using donor sperm, donor egg, surrogacy, gestational carriers, and embryo adoption. This book may be helpful to you as you consider these options. Also, if you are considering donor sperm, the book *Helping the Stork: The Choices and Challenges of Donor Insemination,* by Carol Frost Vercollone, Robert Moss, and Heidi Moss (1997) provides current and relevant information on such issues as deciding between an anonymous and a known donor, dealing with significant others, and deciding whether or not to tell the child.

Sometimes, as in the example of Charlie, you can address these concerns without having to reject the option entirely. Having two rather than three embryos transferred during IVF, if you are opposed to selective reduction, is an example of this. If your concerns are based on cultural or religious beliefs or expectations, you may find it helpful to consult an elder in your community or a respected member of your faith. It can also be helpful to read about how other couples have sorted through these difficult and complex issues. Ellen Glazer and Susan Cooper's book *Without Child: Experiencing and Resolving Infertility* (1988) is filled with short stories, essays, and poems written by ordinary couples who have walked in your shoes and have found their way through these very challenging issues.

Finally, if you find yourselves stuck on the horns of an ethical dilemma and can't seem to work it through, you may find it helpful to see a counselor in your area who has specialized knowledge about the available fertility options. Your fertility center should be able to provide names of qualified counselors, or you can contact the national office of RESOLVE for the names of fertility counselors in your area (see Resources).

Assessing the Importance of Genetic Ties

One of the most basic assumptions that we grow up with is the belief that we have control over our fertility, and another basic assumption is that the child or children we eventually raise will share our genetic history. Unless you knew from an early age that you might never be able to produce children, you probably believed the option to have your own genetic offspring was available to you. As I said before, when you make the choice to parent with someone, you usually have a desire to see the things you love about your partner reflected in your child. Even if there is a history of mental or physical health problems in your families, you probably feel some comfort in knowing what these are. Indeed, we all make some sense of who we are as people, based on our understanding of our genetic histories. Knowing the traits, strengths, and characteristics that tend to run in your respective gene pools helps put yourselves and your identities into context. It gives you a sense of generational continuity.

When faced with infertility, you are forced to confront your basic beliefs and values about the importance of genetic ties. Each time you face a new treatment option, you and your partner have to ask yourselves how important parenting is to you both. If "very important" is the answer, the next question is, "How important is it for us to have our own biological child?" You will find yourself faced with this question repeatedly throughout the process of diagnosis and treatment, especially when you are contemplating third-party reproductive options such as using donor eggs or sperm. You'll also find yourselves asking this question when considering other parenting options like adoption or foster parenting.

This is often a very difficult question and you may be surprised by how strongly you feel about your child being genetically related to you. In North American culture, the importance of genetic ties is strongly reinforced. Our language is a reflection of this. For example, in cases of children who are adopted as infants, it is common for people to refer to the biological parents of the child as the "real" or "natural" parents. Even though the adoptive parents assume the full responsibility of raising the child, our language infers that their claim is somehow not as legitimate as that of the persons who provided the genetic material. The same is true in the case of egg or embryo donation. The gestational mother—the woman who receives the donation, and in whose body the fetus develops—may not consider herself, or be considered by others, to be the child's "real" mother. Couples who are considering the option of using donor sperm frequently worry that the child will have a closer bond with the female partner, the biological parent, and that the child may even want to seek out the donor at some point in the future.

Andrea and Doug went through just this struggle. Everyone who knew Andrea believed she'd make a great mother. She was a "natural" with kids and looked forward to have a large family. However, shortly after she married Doug, Andrea's older sister gave birth to a severely disabled child. Genetic testing indicated a chromosomal abnormality carried by the women in Andrea's family. Andrea and Doug were devastated by this news. They agreed that they were not willing to risk passing the disorder on to their offspring. Their parenting options were to use donor eggs or adopt a child. Doug's older brother, Bob, and his wife, Lori, offered to provide Andrea and Doug with oocytes. They had two young children of their own and weren't planning to have any more. According to Lori, she had eggs that were being "wasted" every month and she couldn't think of two people who would make better parents than Andrea and Doug. She and Bob were clear in their minds and hearts that these were "just eggs" and that Andrea would be the child's "real mother" if treatment was successful. Andrea was very grateful to Lori and Bob, but before she could accept their offer Andrea had to work through her feelings of loss as well as her fears that the child would later reject her, because although she would be the child's birth mother she would not be his or her genetic mother.

As you are contemplating the importance of genetic ties at each stage of the treatment process, you may find it helpful to ask yourselves the following critical question: Can we love a child who is not genetically related to us? If the answer to that question is "yes," then you've taken a big step toward opening up the possibility of other parenting options. You will still have to deal with the many losses associated with not having your own biological children. You may also continue to pursue treatment options that afford you the chance of having a child who is genetically related to at least one of you. And should you elect to consider adoption or the use of donated sperm or eggs, you will have to work through your fears and concerns about problems that might arise for the child as a consequence of his or her genetic background.

If your answer to the question is "I'm not sure," "We're not sure," "I can but my partner can't," or "My partner can but I can't," then you're probably not ready to consider adoption or third-party reproductive options. While you don't want to close off any of the available parenting options prematurely, you should not go ahead with third-party reproductive treatment or adoption unless both you and your partner can answer yes to this question. No one knows for certain how they're going to feel when they bring home the child they have created or adopted. Some degree of uncertainty is realistic and understandable. Like parenthood itself, making the commitment to loving and raising a child who is not genetically related to you requires a certain leap of faith—that you're up to the challenge and that you're capable of loving the child irrespective of your genetic differences. If you can't yet make that leap, that's okay. As described in the example of Ted and Susan in chapter 2, the costs of going ahead when you're not ready are even greater than electing not to pursue a particular option that you're not yet comfortable with.

If the answer to the question is "definitely not," you have the answer you need at this point to make decisions you can live with. If you have time to let things settle and to reopen this issue at a later point in the process, then take the time you need. If not, and one of you wants to go ahead with a particular treatment or parenting option but the other doesn't feel comfortable doing so, you may need some professional assistance to help you work through your differences on this issue. The suggestions in the next section may also be useful if you and your partner are deadlocked on what to do, or not to do, next.

Deadlocked: Negotiating Decisions with Your Partner

Partners frequently have different beliefs about what they should do next. Should we consider the treatment option being recommended? Is it time to pursue other parenting options? Have we done enough? Should we abandon the whole thing and just get on with our lives without children? Disagreements over these important issues are very common, because although infertility is a couple's issue, the reality is that each of you experiences infertility in a different way and on a different emotional schedule. You may not be equally invested in parenthood, or in having your own genetic offspring. You may have different levels of readiness to pursue certain treatment or parenting options.

Whatever your specific situation, being deadlocked with your partner on such an important life issue can add tremendously to the already considerable stresses of infertility. You may find yourself full of anger and rage if you feel your partner is blocking your chance to have a child or is insisting on pursuing an option you aren't comfortable with.

Thirty-six-year-old Sue and forty-five-year-old Marty found themselves at odds with each other over the issue of having children. When they met, Sue was pretty clear that having children wasn't something she needed in her life. She had never felt any desire to be a mother and was very satisfied with her life and her career. Marty, on the other hand, really wanted kids. He was willing to take primary responsibility for the child rearing, especially in the early years, so Sue finally agreed to throw away her birth control pills. When their efforts to have a child weren't successful and Marty was diagnosed with a low sperm count, Sue reluctantly agreed to several cycles of intrauterine inseminations (IUI) with Marty's washed sperm, and despite her intense opposition to taking medications of any sort, she even agreed to ovulation induction. When this was unsuccessful, Marty wanted to try IVF. Sue, however, refused. Although she didn't want to deny Marty the opportunity to become a father, she was not willing to go through the ordeal of taking even larger doses of hormone medications and the invasive procedures of IVF. Marty was sensitive to Sue's concerns but he felt that she was being unreasonable and selfish in refusing to try IVF even once. It took them several sessions of counseling to work through their deadlock on this issue. Eventually they decided to try one IVF cycle, agreeing that if this was unsuccessful they'd abandon their treatment efforts.

If you find yourself in a situation like Sue and Marty's, you may find the suggestions below helpful as you attempt to work through your differences and try to make the kinds of decisions you both can live with.

Try to See This as an Opportunity

These differences are normal, and in fact they can be very helpful. First, they force you both to slow down the process and not jump prematurely into the next round of treatment. This means that instead of immediately deciding to use the cryopreserved embryos left over from your failed IVF cycle, you give your body and your emotions some time to recover. Or it may mean that, instead of immediately using donor sperm after a failed ICSI cycle, you both have some time to deal with the loss of not being able to produce a child who shares both of your genetic histories. In taking some time to regroup and heal, you're more likely to gain the perspective and energy you need to make more satisfying choices about what to do next.

Also, bumping up against your partner's resistance to, or insistence on, a particular treatment or parenting option can result in more clarity for both of you as you decide what you really need to do next, and why. It forces you both to take a good, hard look at your beliefs, values, and motivations. In discussing and debating your individual perspectives on these very important issues, you may well find that you end up making more informed and satisfying decisions together.

Be Clear on Who or What the Enemy Is

When you desperately want something that is of great importance to you, and you feel your partner is blocking you in your
efforts to reach your goal, it is easy to begin to see your partner as the
enemy. However, this belief is neither true nor useful. The enemy
that you're fighting is infertility and *you're both on the same side in this
battle*. Try not to lose sight of the fact that you're in this together. You
are both headed down this road because you have agreed that parenthood is something you want and need in your lives.

As you face obstacle after obstacle, you're both forced to repeatedly reconsider your motivations and desires for parenthood. You're
forced to ask yourselves over and over again, "Do we still want to be
parents, and at what cost?" You're not always going to come up with
the same answers as your partner, and you certainly won't come up
with the same answer on the same schedule. But that doesn't mean
you're not on the same side. It just means that you both need to take
time to work through why you're feeling the need to keep pushing
ahead, or why you're feeling some resistance to doing so. It means
that the two of you need to step back, regroup, and strategize your
next course of action.

Know Yourself

As I discussed earlier in this chapter, it is important to know
your decision-making style. When dealing with differences between
your desires and those of your partner, knowing yourself is also
really critical. If you're wishing to pursue a particular treatment
option but your partner is not, you need to ask yourself why you
need to do this. Is it because you believe that this new treatment has
a good chance of working? Is it because your doctors have learned
something from your last treatment cycle and feel that they can make
this one more successful? Is it because you feel you can't walk away
until you've tried everything medicine has to offer? Is it because
you're afraid of having regrets later? Is it because you can't face the
uncertainty of another process, like adoption? Is it because you're
afraid to let go of the dream of having your own biological child? Is it
because a life without children wouldn't be tolerable?

On the other hand, if you're not willing to undertake a treatment your physician recommends, or you want to move on to considering other parenting options but your partner does not, you need
to sort out why you feel this way. Perhaps you don't believe the

treatment would work. Perhaps you're not willing to put your body through the odeal that comes with taking all the drugs. Perhaps you're afraid of having to face one more failure. Perhaps you're concerned that your marriage won't survive the stress of another treatment cycle. Perhaps you're concerned that if you use all of your financial resources on treatment and it doesn't work, there won't be enough money left over for adoption.

All of these concerns are legitimate. None of the options are easy. It's also not easy to abandon your hopes and dreams of going through a pregnancy and childbirth together, of creating a family with your partner. But knowing why you feel the way you do is an important first step in sorting this out with your partner.

Be Respectful of Your Partner's Feelings

Just as you have your own beliefs, needs, fears, and investments in this process, so does your partner. And just as you want your partner to be respectful and considerate of your feelings regarding which course of action you want to pursue next, you also need to be respectful of his or hers. This is often easier said than done, especially when you feel committed to your option, and it seems like your partner is the only thing standing in your way.

When you start to feel this way, you need to step back and ask yourself what it is that you need from your partner. Usually, you need to feel heard and understood, even if she or he doesn't agree with your position. Your partner has the same needs. If you both feel that your perspectives are understood and respected, you have a much better chance of coming to some agreement on what to do next, and of finding a way to compromise.

Communicate Clearly and Directly

It's fine to talk about understanding your own needs, beliefs, and preferences, and about being respectful of your partner's rights to his or her beliefs and feelings. However, if you're going to make any headway in solving your differences you'll need to be able to communicate with each other in a way that allows you both to feel heard and understood. Some basic rules of communication can be helpful in this regard.

1. *Take ownership of your own stuff.* Blaming your partner for how you feel will not help you resolve this impasse. For example,

if you say, "You're keeping me from having the most important thing in my life," or "You're forcing me to do something
I don't believe in," your partner will likely feel attacked and
become defensive, growing even more set in his or her own
position. However, if you say, "I realize that you don't necessarily feel the same way, but I need you to understand how
important being a parent is to me," or "I know you're comfortable with this option, but I need some time to sort out
why it doesn't feel right for me," your partner will be less
likely to become defensive. The difference between these two
approaches is subtle, but important. In the first, you're plac-
ing blame. In the second, you're respecting your partner's
rights to his or her feelings, while also taking ownership of,
and clarifying, your own position.

2. *Be specific about the decision you're trying to make.* It is easy to
lose sight of your goals in general discussions about rights
and principles and values—issues that rarely can be resolved.
On the other hand, sorting through a specific decision (for
example, "Do we try a cycle of IVF or do we move directly to
donor sperm?") is much more manageable, and solvable.

3. *Keep the issue contained.* When you're deadlocked over an
important issue such as whether or not you're going to keep
trying to have a child, the stakes are very high. You may feel
like you're being betrayed by your partner, and you may
even question whether the two of you should be together,
and whether you have the same values and want the same
things in life. These thoughts and feelings can bleed into all
aspects of your relationship and wind up pushing you even
farther apart. By staying focused on the specific decision to
be made, you'll have a better chance of maintaining your perspective and your connection to each other, and of working it
through together.

4. *Give each other space to consider and respond.* In all relationships
there are "hot" issues—issues that are so important to one or
both of you that just talking about them ignites tremendous
tension between you. How to respond to your infertility can
certainly be one of those hot issues. It can be very helpful to
find ways to communicate your feelings and perspectives to
your partner that allows him or her to hear and reflect on
them, without having to immediately respond. Try putting
your feelings in writing, using "I" statements (e.g., "I'm feel-

ing frustrated that the doctor's can't tell us why we are unable to get pregnant), and ask your partner to read what you have written and take some time before responding. This method can be a very effective way to take some of the heat out of the debate. It can also be helpful to set specific times to discuss the decision in question, and agree to talk about the decision only during those times. As a result the issues get addressed and discussed, without every interaction between you and your partner deteriorating into a battle.

Up Against the Clock: Responding to the Pressures of Time

Decision making can be challenging enough when you're trying to produce a child with medical assistance, but when your time is limited by biology, it can be even more difficult to make rational and satisfying decisions. It may be fine to talk about stepping back from treatment and taking time to consider your options carefully. But when you're pushing forty and you feel like your eggs are aging by the minute, it's hard not to panic. Even if you weren't panicked before you started fertility treatments, the whole climate of fertility centers turns up the heat considerably. These are far from the best circumstances for making informed decisions. You will do well, however, to keep in mind that your fertility status is unlikely to change dramatically overnight. Even if you're thirty-four and you've heard that the odds of success are lower for women over thirty-five, or you're thirty-nine and are about to enter the poor prognosis range of women over forty, chances are that you have a few weeks or months to make a decision without compromising your odds of success. The same holds for sperm counts. Sperm parameters can change marginally on a daily basis, but dramatic changes in a short period of time are unlikely.

Perhaps your sense of urgency isn't based on medical statistics and prognoses. Rather, it may have to do with your personal time frame for starting your family, a time frame that may already have been pushed up much farther than you'd like. Or perhaps you're like many couples and feel that it's too late to start a family after a certain age. Again, it is important to remember that, although these dates are important benchmarks for you personally, they don't necessarily relate to your fertility—something that you're probably beginning to realize isn't under your control anyway. Or maybe your feeling of urgency comes from the desire to have some resolution to this whole fertility issue, because you're tired of having your lives on hold.

Rather than driving yourself crazy with the pressure to make quick decisions, take a look at the source of this pressure. If it's based on a schedule you and your partner have set for yourselves, then try to adjust your timeline. Specific deadlines set in advance can add a lot of unnecessary pressure to a situation that already has enough stress. If you find that your sense of urgency comes from concerns about a decline in your fertility or your chances of success, you need to check these assumptions out with your physician. Don't be afraid to ask whether it will make a difference in your chances if you decide to wait a few months to make your decision. If the pressure your feeling comes from a desire for resolution and a need to take your lives off hold, then the suggestions in chapter 7 might help you to move forward in other areas of your lives, and to avoid making treatment and parenting decisions under pressure.

Finally, if you're a woman, don't expect your partner to feel the same sense of pressure that you do, unless he's been diagnosed with a male factor problem. As noted in chapter 1, men don't usually feel the same pressure to parent that women do, partially because they aren't faced with the same biological time limitations, and because their social worlds aren't as focused on raising children as women's are. They may not even begin to feel the same pressure to become fathers until they're in their forties. So talk about why you're feeling pressure to move forward. Try to give yourselves a bit of time and space to recoup, to find out how you feel about your choices, and to carefully consider what next step is right for you both.

Selecting a Fertility Specialist: "Whom Can We Trust?"

The specialist into whose hands you put your bodies, your hopes, and your trust plays a very important part in your experience of infertility. Whatever the eventual outcome of treatment, it will be easier to deal with if you feel you've been treated with honesty, respect, compassion, and competence. This is especially the case if medical testing doesn't result in a diagnosis, or if your treatment efforts don't result in a pregnancy. When you have a good relationship with your health-care providers, you'll find it easier to cope with your feelings about your infertility and medical experiences, if the treatments fail. Of course, if the treatments succeed, you'll likely be grateful irrespective of your experience with the people who helped you realize your dreams.

Selecting a fertility specialist, then, is an important decision. When making this decision you need to take several things into account.

- *Specialization.* Some general practitioners and most gynecologists treat fertility-related problems with a fair degree of success. Most can conduct the basic medical workup and can intervene in situations that require relatively minor medical intervention (such as treating a mild ovulatory irregularity with clomiphene), or in the case of the gynecologist, some fertility-promoting surgical problems. However, when it comes to the diagnosis and treatment of more complex fertility issues, a physician who specializes in reproductive medicine would be indicated. Your general practitioner or health insurer may be able to recommend a reproductive endocrinologist in your area. You can also obtain this information from the American Society for Reproductive Medicine, RESOLVE, or, in Canada, the Infertility Awareness Association or the Infertilty Network. (see Resources).

- *Location.* Fertility testing and treatments usually take up a tremendous amount of time. When you're considering any of the advanced reproductive technologies, you'll be asked to do repeated blood tests and ultrasounds, semen analyses, and a number of other procedures. For this reason, you'll want to choose a specialist who is located close to your workplace or home. If your specialist is located in another county or on the other side of a large city, just traveling to and from the medical office can add pressure to an already very stressful situation. These difficulties, and your financial expenses, can be even greater if your specialist is in another city and you have to pay for travel and extended hotel stays during the diagnostic or treatment process. If you must choose a specialist who is in another city, it may be wise to select one in a city where you have close friends or family with whom you can stay during treatment.

- *Track record.* During the course of fertility investigations and treatments, your financial and emotional investment in trying to have a child will likely be quite high. It is important, then, that you feel confident in your health-care provider's ability to assist you. One way to assess this is to ask questions about the number of times the specialist has performed the procedure in question, and about the rates of success she or he has achieved with this treatment on people of the same age and diagnostic status. Most specialists expect to be asked these questions and are comfortable providing you with this information.

- *Personal fit.* Every specialist has his or her own style of communicating and working with patients. Some are very gregarious and optimistic, instilling confidence that you're in the right hands and that they can help you and your partner have a baby. Others are very factual, shooting from the hip, so to speak. They may not always tell you what you wish to hear, but their demeanor tells you that they're giving you all the facts, so that you have the information you need to make whatever decision that is best for you. Still others are very quiet and clinical, perhaps not making much eye contact with you, just giving you the information on what they recommend and what they're willing or able to do to treat your fertility problem. Some personal styles will work better for you than others, so try to take this into account when selecting a specialist. You need to choose someone whom you're comfortable working with.

Trusting Your Instincts

Above all else it is important to trust your instincts. Whether you're selecting a fertility specialist, considering a treatment option, or picking a donor, there is a point at which it is important to listen to your intuition—the part that, deep down, knows what you need to do.

To a certain degree, decision making is a logical process, and it's good to be logical. As noted above, it's also good to be informed. However, decision making is also an intuitive process. You can probably think of decisions you've made in your life that, if you were being completely logical, you'd never have made. In fact, some people even say that, given the huge financial costs of raising a child to adulthood, not to mention the loss of personal freedom that comes with parenthood, choosing to have children is an illogical decision. And yet it is a choice most people make.

Indeed, as you face a particular treatment decision or parenting option, when you and your partner sit down with your list of pros and cons you may find that the list of reasons not to pursue this option is much longer than the list of reasons to go ahead—and yet you still decide you need to "go for it." Over the years I've heard many couples say that they know they've made the right decision about a particular donor or a particular treatment. As long as they've assessed all the available information and taken a bit of time to let their decision settle, I always encourage them to trust their instincts. I strongly encourage you to do this as well. Trusting your instincts is like trusting yourself. Trusting yourself isn't always easy, especially when you're feeling like a failure because you can't get pregnant or because your sperm isn't viable, but it is important. It helps you feel that you have some power in a very challenging situation. It is also critical in ensuring that, whatever the outcome, you won't have regrets.

How Much Is Enough?

This is undoubtedly one of the most difficult questions you'll face while trying to make treatment and parenting decisions. It is very complex, so much so I've devoted chapter 8 to how to sort through this issue. It is important not to decide in advance to end your quest for parenthood simply because you have tried a particular treatment option or reached a particular birthday. As I said above, you can't know early in this process just how far you and your partner will need to go, or be willing to go, in your efforts to produce a child. You won't know that until you get there, and even then it may not be entirely clear-cut.

It can be helpful for you to set a *tentative* time frame within which you hope to finish pursuing treatment, or by the end of which you hope to begin the adoption process. By leaving your time frame open, you'll allow yourselves some flexibility to alter your plans or take extra time when you need to, rather than feeling forced to stick to a rigid schedule.

4

Coping with the Stresses of Medical Testing and Treatment

Anyone who has been through infertility will tell you that it is a very difficult, challenging, and stressful experience. Some have even said that it is a worse crisis than going through a divorce or the death of a parent. Couples are usually grateful that medical science offers a number of procedures for diagnosing and treating infertility. Ironically, however, some of the greatest stress and distress experienced by infertile couples happens during the months or years when they're going through these procedures.

As described in chapter 2, some of the tests and procedures can be expensive, especially the advanced reproductive technologies. You may experience some of the tests and treatments as physically uncomfortable, or even painful. The most private aspects of your lives and bodies are exposed and subjected to medical examination; to make matters worse, despite all of these tests and exams, sometimes no answers can be found that would explain why you aren't getting pregnant, or why a particular treatment cycle wasn't sucessful.

Because treatment can last for months or years, experiencing medical intervention isn't a discrete event. The stresses are often prolonged, wearing down your personal resources over time. The longer it takes to find answers, the greater the stress and emotional distress. As Kathryn, a forty-year-old sales associate who, with her partner

Jack, spent eight years involved in fertility treatments, says, fertility interventions just aren't like other medical procedures.

> *People just don't realize that infertility treatment is different. It's not a factual, clear-cut kind of medical experience. You don't just have an operation and everything is better—it's all fixed. It goes on and on and on. Even if it works once, you still have to go through it again if you want a bigger family. And it wears you down. It's much more emotional than it is medical, as far as I'm concerned.*

Finding effective ways to handle the ongoing stresses of medical treatment is the focus of this chapter.

Although a lot has been written about coping, there really isn't one right or healthy way to respond to stress just as there isn't one right way to deal with infertility or with medical testing and treatment. However, there are certain strategies that other couples have found helpful in their efforts to deal with fertility treatments. These are discussed below. Not all of them will work for you or your partner, so try to select the ones that fit best with your own coping styles. Before discussing these strategies, it is important to first define coping.

What Is Coping?

Coping is an active, adaptive response to a perceived threat, in this case the threat of being childless. Both infertility and medical treatment can present a threat to your body, life goals, dreams of the future, beliefs and expectations, emotional equilibrium, and relationship with your partner. The experience of being infertile and going through repeated medical tests and procedures will likely threaten to deplete your emotional and personal resources. In response, you'll try to do things to overcome the stress and reduce the threat:

- You may respond *cognitively* by arming yourself with relevant information about infertility diagnosis and treatment, or by setting concrete goals for your pursuit of treatment.

- You may respond *emotionally* by minimizing the severity of the situation or finding ways to release your frustration and express your feelings.

- You may respond *behaviorally* by practicing relaxation and pain management techniques, or by actively pursuing other parenting options while undergoing treatment.

- You may find yourself responding *psychologically* by defending against the feelings and pain of treatment and infertility by immersing yourself in work or withdrawing from social contacts and activities you enjoy.

Your responses will depend on how severe you perceive the threat to be, and on your available coping resources. The greater the threat, the stronger your instinct will be to respond in ways to reduce it.

Understanding Your Coping Styles

How you cope with infertility and with medical testing and treatment will be the result of a number of factors: your personality, your outlook on life, and how you've learned to deal with threatening situations. In fact, looking back at a specific event in your life that was especially stressful can be a good way to assess your coping style. If you feel you successfully weathered that event, knowing this can give you very useful information about the personal resources that you have. Many of these resources can serve you well when you are dealing with infertility treatments. Although infertility may feel like one of the worst things you've faced in your life, it may be comforting to know that you've coped effectively in the past with other very difficult and challenging situations and can probably handle this one too.

Each of us tends to cope with stress in characteristic ways. Your coping style may be very similar to that of your partner, or it may be quite different. Your styles might complement or conflict with one another. Let's take a closer look at some of the more common coping patterns.

Optimism versus Pessimism

You may be an optimist or a pessimist—you may be the type who sees the cup as half full or the type who sees the cup as half empty. If you are the kind of person who tends to look at situations and life more optimistically—someone who sees the cup half full—when faced with a threat like infertility your tendency will be to frame it as a hurdle that, with perseverance and effort, can be over-come. If you are more of a pessimist—someone who sees the cup half empty—you'll likely frame it as a potentially insurmountable hurdle. When interpreting treatment success rates, if you're a pessimist you'll focus on the 80 percent chance of treatment not being successful. If you're an optimist, you'll focus on the 20 percent chance of success.

When it comes to handling infertility, you and your partner may both be optimists. Although you'll struggle with the pain of failed treatment cycles, you'll probably recover a bit quicker, pulling each other up and maintaining hope that something will eventually work. If you're both pessimists, rebounding from a failed treatment cycle will be more difficult. It may be harder to find the emotional energy to keep on pursuing solutions to your childlessness.

Interestingly, most infertile couples I've worked with seem to embody a combination of optimism and pessimism. It's not at all unusual for one partner to be very optimistic and "positive" about their chances of being successful on their next treatment cycle, irre-spective of the odds, while the other partner seems to be less certain about the outcome. It's not that they aren't equally hopeful that treat-ment will work—no one puts themselves and their bodies through all of this unless they believe they have *some* chance of success. It's just that one partner—often the woman—feels a need to protect herself or himself from feeling devastated if treatment fails. In a sense, keep-ing their optimism in check is a way in which that particular partner copes with the stress of treatment.

Couples sometimes struggle with this difference in their levels of optimism, with the more optimistic partner fearing that the less optimistic one isn't as committed to treatment or isn't giving treat-ment his or her best effort. Those who believe in the power of posi-tive thinking fear that a negative attitude will somehow keep the treatment from being successful. Certainly positive thinking can be a very useful way for some people to deal with treatment, but *there is no conclusive, scientific evidence to support the belief that positive thinking will affect pregnancy rates.* If positive thinking could improve the chances of conception, almost all couples would become pregnant right away, since at the beginning most couples are quite optimistic about having a child together, and sex is still a positive part of their relationship.

Whatever your characteristic style of coping is, try to strike a balance, individually, and between you and your partner while you are dealing with the ongoing stresses of treatment. If your tendency is to look on the negative side, try to identify some of the positive aspects of the course of action you've decided to pursue. For example, forty-two-year-old Alice and her fifty-three-year-old husband, Steve, knew they had pretty poor odds of achieving a pregnancy. Given Alice's age and Steve's deteriorating sperm count, even if they did manage to become pregnant through in vitro fertilization (IVF), they would face an increased chance of miscarriage and a significant risk that their child would suffer from a chromosomal abnormality. On the positive side, however, both Alice and Steve felt that by going through IVF they would achieve closure by having done everything possible to produce a child together.

The coping response that seems to work best for most people during treatment is "cautious optimism." You want to be optimistic enough to have the energy you'll need for pursuing treatment, but not so optimistic that you'll find yourself emotionally devastated if treatment doesn't work.

Internal versus External Sense of Control

How you handle medical treatment will also have to do with the amount of control you feel you have over your decisions and the treatment process. If you feel you have some control over what treatments you undertake and when they happen, it will be much easier to weather the ups and downs of treatment than it will be if you feel that these factors are out of your hands. If your tendency is to assume that you can't effect change in your life, or that you are powerless to achieve the things in life that are important to you, then treatment will be far more stressful and you'll have more difficulty coping.

Having said this, I want to point out that the relationship between control and coping with infertility is not entirely straightforward. The issue of control can be very sticky when it comes to infertility because unrealistic expectations about your ability to control the outcome of treatment can lead you to feel responsible if treatment fails. So believing you have control over the outcome can be problematic. However, believing you have some control over the process can be a very effective way of managing infertility treatments.

Whatever your usual style, an important way to cope with the stresses of treatment, then, will be to identify the things you do have control over, however small or minor they may seem. This might mean asking to be kept fully informed about the purposes and results of the tests, the available treatment options, and when these treatments can occur. It might mean asking your physician if it is okay to stop taking your basal body temperature (BBT) once ovulation has been confirmed. It may mean requesting that you be allowed to collect your semen sample in a less clinical and uncomfortable environment than the medical office. It may mean asking to specify the number of embryos that are transferred during an IVF cycle, within the limits of what is considered good medical practice.

There is no shortage of decisions to make as you negotiate the diagnostic and treatment process, and taking control over the course of your treatment can go a long way in helping you cope. Before you begin any treatment, take the time to identify the things you can choose. Then decide which of these things will help diminish the stress of the procedure, and act on those decisions.

Emotion-Focused versus Problem-Focused Coping

Another difference in the way people cope with difficult and stressful situations is in how they tend to respond: either by venting their frustrations, fears, and feelings, or by trying to fix the problem. This is one area where men and women frequently differ.

Because men are socialized to be in control and take charge of situations, it is not at all uncommon for them to move into a problem-solving mode when confronting infertility and treatment. If this is your style of coping, you may seem almost unemotional in your efforts to process information on the various treatment options, their costs, and their respective probabilities of successful outcome. Talking about the stress or injustice of the situation may seem to you like wasting energy.

Women, on the other hand, tend to rely on more emotion-focused methods when dealing with infertility and medical treatment. If this is your style, you may find that you need to vent—expressing your frustration, anger, pain, and distress. You know it won't change your situation, but expressing yourself makes you feel better. It helps relieve some of the tension. And when it comes to making treatment decisions, all the facts may point to the futility of trying another treatment cycle, but you may just feel that's what you need to do, even if it doesn't make sense to someone else.

Problem-focused coping can be very effective in many situations in life, especially those that are controllable, which is the case with some of the aspects of the fertility treatment *process*. Emotion-focused coping can also be very effective, especially in handling situations and stressors that are uncontrollable, such as the *outcome* of treatment. Ideally, a combination of both approaches can be particularly useful in coping with fertility treatments. Try to problem-solve about the treatment process and figure out what will make this most manageable for you. Then when you need to address your anxieties and fears about the outcome, make a point of finding healthy outlets for your feelings; these outlets may be through physical activities (e.g., running, sports, dance, yoga), words (e.g., talking with others, writing in a journal), or other forms of expression (e.g., painting, playing or listening to music).

Turning Inward versus Reaching Outward

Another difference in the way people cope with stress is their tendency to keep their problems to themselves or to reach out to others to help share their burden. Again, neither style is better than the other in coping with infertility, and, again, men and women tend to differ in their preferred styles. Men tend not to share their infertility struggles with anyone other than their partners, especially in the early stages of treatment. Women, on the other hand, often find comfort in sharing their struggles and distress with close friends or family members, especially in the early stages of treatment. This pattern often changes to one of increasing isolation for both members of the couple in the middle and later stages of treatment, followed by greater sharing with others once treatment is over.

The issue of whether to reach out for support, and whether others can truly be supportive when you're going through infertility treatments (especially if they've never experienced infertility themselves) is a difficult one. Chapter 6 is devoted to addressing this issue more thoroughly. What is most important to note here is that, whether your preferred style is to turn inward or reach outward, you'll need to talk about this issue with your partner and come to some compromise regarding the degree to which you will share your struggles with others. For example, if your partner wants to keep this issue completely confidential but you would get a lot of relief from talking about your fertility struggles with supportive friends or family members, you may agree to limit your sharing to just one or two people whom both you and your partner feel you can trust. If you don't come to some agreement, this issue can cause problems in your relationship and add significantly to the stresses of treatment.

Gender Differences in the Experience of Treatment

Another difference in the way couples cope with fertility treatments is in their degree of involvement in the actual treatment process. As described in chapter 2, much of the focus of medical intervention is on the female partner. Because women's reproductive biology is more complex than men's, women tend to undergo more diagnostic testing. Women are usually the ones who are prescribed fertility drugs. Women are the ones who undergo repeated ultrasounds and gynecological procedures.

This does not mean that men aren't also subjected to difficult and painful tests and procedures, especially in cases where a male factor problem is diagnosed. Testicular biopsies, varicocele repairs, and vasectomy reversals often cause considerable physical discomfort, and repeated semen analyses are pretty uncomfortable for many men. However, even in cases of male factor infertility, the female partner is the one who carries the pregnancy and, as a consequence, her body and hormonal functioning are still a central focus of medical testing and intervention. Also, the outcome of treatment usually plays itself out in the woman's body, often resulting in feelings of accountability and failure on the woman's part, even if the problem is with her partner's sperm.

These differences in the experience of medical testing and treatment often mean that women feel more ongoing stress and distress than do their partners. While both men and women may find it difficult to cope with being infertile, it is often the woman's emotional resources that are severely put to the test on an ongoing basis during treatment. This is why, when a couple are trying to decide whether to pursue a treatment option such as in vitro fertilization, the man will often defer to his partner to make the final decision since it is her body and her life that undergo the greatest disruption during treatment.

You need to take these differences into consideration, when you're learning to understand your stress reactions and coping responses and those of your partner. Also, you need to remember that the experience of undergoing medical fertility treatments is not just physical, it is also emotional. If treatment fails, it is very common to feel that it's somehow your fault or your partner's fault—that one of you did something wrong or didn't handle the stress appropriately. This only adds to the distress of infertility. Let's take a closer look, then, at the relationship between stress and infertility.

The Relationship between Stress and Infertility

There has been a lot of speculation and discussion over the years about the relationship between stress and infertility. As I pointed out in chapter 1, when medical answers couldn't be found to explain why a couple weren't able to get or maintain a viable pregnancy, it was assumed by mental health professionals that the woman must be doing something psychologically to block her fertility. Although this belief has been proven to be false, the assumption that stress, or positive or negative thoughts, can have an impact on fertility is still very common. It is the basis for much of the unsolicited advice you've probably received from other people explaining why you aren't getting pregnant, telling you that you could get pregnant if you just tried hard enough, lowered your stress levels, and learned to relax. It is also the reason that, after an embryo transfer, many women try to do everything they can—from eating good foods, to thinking positive thoughts, to staying off work and off their feet for two weeks—to ensure that a pregnancy will "take."

The reality, however, is that we really don't know a lot about the relationship between stress and fertility. There has been some recent research suggesting that women who join stress-reduction therapy groups during treatment may have a greater chance of conceiving. But the results of this research are still inconclusive (Domar 1997). As yet the research studies don't explain why some women become pregnant following stress reduction training but others do not. It is known that women in very stressful situations sometimes become pregnant (e.g., during a rape), and that women who desperately do not want to get pregnant sometimes do. Also, all of the available research supports the fact that women who undergo fertility treatments experience significantly more stress than women who do not. Infertility and fertility treatments are very stressful. Despite this fact, approximately 50 percent of all women who go through fertility investigations and treatment end up becoming pregnant (Corson 1999).

At this point in time, the relationship between stress and fertility is very unclear. If you're going through treatment, the best approach may be to do what you need to do to keep yourself sane and healthy. If you've had embryos transferred and you're doing something strenuous, like lifting a box or riding a bike, and you ask yourself several times whether you should be doing this, then it is probably best not to. It may have no effect whatsoever on whether you become pregnant, but, if you're like most women, if the treatment fails you'll look back at the cycle and wonder if it was because of something you did or didn't do, because you didn't have the right attitude, or because you were too "stressed out." So it's probably better to err on the side of caution. Just don't assume you have control over the outcome. Just as you didn't choose to be infertile, you don't have control over your fertility—only how you cope with it.

Coping with Your New Identity as Patient

One of the first things you have to get accustomed to when you begin fertility investigations is the fact that, whatever your identity may be in the rest of your life, once you enter the doors of a fertility clinic you become a patient. You become identified by your medical problem or diagnostic status, and you spend a large amount of time waiting for medical and counseling appointments, phone calls, blood tests, ultrasounds, test results, and treatment procedures.

The medical staff are the people with the expertise, and you become the recipient of their wisdom. The playing field is far from level, because you and your partner are the ones with the problem and they are the ones with the power to fix the problem. You're vulnerable, because these people are the conduit between your dreams of having a child and permanent biological childlessness. They are powerful and you feel powerless. This sense of powerlessness is heightened by the fact that you spend a fair bit of time during the treatment process lying on your back, half dressed, with your feet in stirrups and your legs spread, or sitting in a little room with some erotic magazines and a small sterile bottle.

The medical staff may be very caring and compassionate. But that doesn't change the fact that you're anxious, uncertain, and fearful. You are relying on these people, and on medical science, to help you achieve one of the most important goals of your life. No matter how competent you feel in the world of work or in other aspects of your life, when you walk into this type of medical situation you lose some of your sense of control and agency. You take on the role of patient, which can make it hard for you to communicate your needs and assert your rights. So, what are your rights as a patient?

- You have the right to be treated with respect and courtesy.

- You have the right to be given accurate diagnostic information.

- You have a right to receive detailed information about the available treatment options and their likelihood of success given your particular circumstances.

- You have the right to get a second opinion.

- You have a right to be fully informed about costs and procedures before starting treatment.

- You have a right to receive information about the medical health and background of the donor, when you are using donor eggs, sperm, or embryos.

- Within legal and institutional limits, you have a right to decide the disposition of your sperm, eggs, and embryos.

There are also some things you can do to help yourself feel less vulnerable and powerless during medical testing and treatment. For example, you can bring your own bathrobe when going through treatments so that you don't have to walk around half naked in an open-backed hospital gown. You can insist on having discussions about tests and treatments in your doctor's office, rather than in a procedure room while you're lying down and only half-dressed. You can ask that the medical staff not call or leave messages for you at work regarding your medications or test results. You can ask to have your partner in the room with you while you're going through medical tests and treatment procedures.

These are just some examples of the ways you can reduce your feelings of powerlessness and vulnerability. Although you will still feel like a patient as long as you're involved in this process, asking for small accommodations like these can help make the experience more manageable. Four years of fertility investigations and treatments taught Terry a lot about her needs and how she could ensure that these were met. Her words underscore the value of asserting your rights while you're trying to find solutions to your infertility:

> Be sure to speak up for your own medical rights and needs. Some doctors may not like that . . . so hopefully you get to choose who you want to be your doctor. You didn't choose to be infertile, but you have choices about what you're going to do about it. That's the part that's empowering—that no one can ever take choice away from you—no matter what happens.

Coping with Pain and Discomfort

As well as having to cope with the emotional distress of infertility, you may also find yourself having to cope with some degree of physical distress. Many of the standard diagnostic tests and treatments can cause some physical pain and discomfort. For some women the hysterosalpingogram (HSG), the laparoscopy, the endometrial biopsy, and the egg-retrieval process cause discomfort. Some women also experience headaches, abdominal discomfort, and bloating when taking superovualtion medications. For men, procedures commonly associated with pain and discomfort include testicular biopsy, varicocele repairs, vasectomy reversal, microsurgical epididymal sperm aspiration (MESA), and testicular sperm extraction (TESE).

It is very difficult to know how you are going to react to the various medications and treatments. Every person has a different pain threshold; sometimes a particular procedure results in more discomfort for one person than another because of differences in their reproductive physiology. This being said, the following suggestions may help you to deal with the physical and, to a degree, the psychological, discomforts of testing and treatment.

Progressive Relaxation and Controlled Breathing

When you are tense (and you will most likely be tense when undergoing fertility testing and treatments), you have a tendency to contract your muscles. Your breathing also becomes more rapid and shallow, resulting in the absorption of less oxygen throughout your body. In most situations, this response only increases the likelihood of experiencing pain and discomfort.

However, with some practice, you can train yourself to enter a state of relaxation. You can decrease the tension in your body, and you can slow down and deepen your breathing. When you do, you will help to initiate what is commonly known as the relaxation response. This response originates in the brain, specifically the hypothalamus. When it occurs, it is associated with a generalized decrease in sympathetic nervous system activity. As a result, not only will you feel calmer, which will help with your stress and anxiety, but you likely won't feel as much pain.

A number of popular books and audio tapes are available that can help you learn to relax while going through uncomfortable tests and procedures (see Resources). You can also learn quite easily on your own by practicing the following exercise for just a few minutes every day:

> Sit quietly in a room without noise or distractions. Get comfortable, either with your back supported in a chair and your feet resting on the floor, or lying down. Close your eyes and turn

your attention to your body. Pay attention to how it feels and try to identify where in your body you are carrying the most tension. Don't try to do anything about it—just notice where it is and how it feels. Now, beginning with your toes, first contract the muscles in your toes for three seconds, then release them completely for five seconds. Next, move to the muscles in your feet. Contracting them for three seconds, then releasing them for five seconds. Slowly and deliberately, work your way up your entire body—your calf muscles, your thighs, your abdomen, your buttocks, your chest, your neck, your jaw, your mouth, your eyes, your forehead, your shoulders, your arms, your hands, and finally your fingers. As you do this, be aware of the sensation in your muscles when they are tense and when the tension is released. Once you've completed this part of the exercise, just sit or lie quietly, with all your muscles relaxed, paying attention now to your breathing. Try to take very slow, easy breaths. Concentrate on breathing in through your nose, slowly, to a count of four or five. Then, very, very slowly, release the breath through your mouth, to a count of eight, nine, or ten. Repeat this several times, until you feel calm and peaceful. Stay with this feeling for a few more minutes.

This very simple exercise can be enormously helpful to do during a stressful test or procedure. By allowing your muscles to relax, rather than contract, you are making it easier for the instrument to be inserted, or the sperm or eggs to be extracted. Focusing on your breathing helps distract you from the procedure, and it ensures that more oxygen is available to the rest of your body.

Mental Imagery and Visualization

Imagery and visualizations also can be very effective tools for handling the stress and physical discomforts of treatment. Visualizing or imagining essentially means creating in your mind an image of a situation or scene—in this case, one that calms you and helps you feel more in control of your feelings and reactions. What goes on in your mind has a direct effect on how your body reacts. For example, if you think about an upcoming test such as the HSG or a sperm analysis, and your mind fills with thoughts of how humiliating or painful the experience will be, your body reacts accordingly. You may feel a tightening in your throat or a clenching in your stomach. If, on the other hand, you visualize the upcoming test or procedure as being relatively easy and painless, then your body will respond by staying relaxed. Visualizations and imagery also work during the procedure, allowing you to mentally escape a painful or unpleasant situation by imagining that you are in a place associated with calm, relaxation, and positive feelings.

It's up to you to decide whether you visualize a particular test or procedure as being easy and pain free, or you visualize yourself in a place or situation that is associated with pleasant and relaxing thoughts or memories. Either approach can be effective in dealing with stress and pain. You may find that one comes easier to you than the other, so try practicing both approaches and see which one seems to work best for you. Also, creating mental images and pictures is easier for some people than it is for others. Even if visualizing doesn't come easy to you, try to persevere. You may be surprised to find, after only a bit of practice, that you begin to catch glimpses of the soothing scenes you'd hoped to create in your mind.

As with relaxation exercises, numerous books and tapes are available to help you learn to use your imagination as a tool for stress and pain relief. Some of the more popular ones can be found in the Resources list. However, you may find the exercise below sufficient to get you started. This exercise will help you visualize yourself in a calm, peaceful setting. First select a calm and positive image, perhaps a favorite place or special memory. Next, follow the instructions in the relaxation exercise above and get yourself into a relaxed state. Your ability to visualize will improve when you are in this state because you'll experience alpha brain waves, the brain waves associated with a state of calm and reduced mental activity.

> Once your breathing has slowed and you begin to feel relaxed, clear your mind of all thoughts. Slowly begin to create a peaceful, soothing scene in your mind in explicit detail. For example, if you are in a meadow, allow yourself to see and feel the grass. Touch it. Run your hands and feet over it. Let the blades slip through your fingers. Allow yourself to drink in all the smells—the fragrance of the flowers, the freshness of the air. Pay attention to all the sounds—the song of the birds, the chirping of the crickets, the sound of the wind. Lie down in the grass, or walk through the meadow. Take it all in. Don't miss a single detail. Allow yourself to stay there as long as you like. Thoroughly enjoy the moment—the peacefulness—the calm. Then, when you're ready, slowly bring yourself back to the present. Be aware of your body. Be aware of your breathing. Take a few deep, slow cleansing breaths, then open your eyes.

Once you've practiced this a few times, it will become easier to take yourself to this place, and you'll be able to get there much quicker. When you're going through a stressful or uncomfortable procedure, you can use this new skill to mentally remove yourself from the situation, returning to your body when the test or procedure is over.

Hypnosis

Another very powerful method of pain and stress control is hypnosis. Like the techniques described above, hypnosis has been practiced for centuries. It has long been used by Native American Indians, and it is still practiced in many Eastern cultures. More recently hypnosis has been used to help people cope with fears and phobias, stop smoking, lose weight, and manage acute and chronic pain. It is also very effective for handling the pain of childbirth.

Hypnosis has been described in many different ways: as a trance state, a state of hyper-suggestibility, or an altered state of consciousness. Over the years much has been learned about this powerful and natural technique. Hypnosis appears to be a natural state that combines a state of deep relaxation with heightened awareness and concentration. In pain management, hypnosis is used to allow a person to be aware of what is going on around them and what is happening to them, while being psychologically removed from the pain just enough to not feel overwhelmed by it. When in a hypnotic state, you are aware of what is happening to you, but you are disconnected from the pain or discomfort. You are there, but you are not there.

When it was first practiced by medical and mental health professionals, hypnosis required a specially trained person to induce a trancelike state in a patient, through the power of suggestion. The therapist or healer had the control, and the patient responded to the therapist's commands and instructions, without any will of his or her own. Although many people still seek the assistance of a hypnotherapist to learn this technique, the principles are relatively straightforward and many find them easy to learn on their own. If you decide self-hypnosis might be useful for you, I'd recommend reading any of the books on the subject listed in the Resources section. Once you learn the basic techniques, you can hypnotize yourself, putting yourself into a trancelike state, in order to cope with the pain and stress of treatment.

Distracters

Another effective way of coping with stress and discomfort during medical tests and procedures is to focus your attention on something that distracts you from what is happening. For example, if music calms or distracts you, you might want to bring in your favorite compact disc to listen to during the test or procedure in question. For many years now people have been coping with the stress caused by dental procedures and surgery by using a personal stereo and listening to music instead of the dreaded sound of the dentist's drill. Many fertility centers also encourage their clients to bring in a tape or compact disc that they want to have played during the egg retrieval, for example. You may elect to bring in quiet, peaceful music that helps you float away to a more relaxing setting. Or you may find that tunes with words can better distract you while you're going through a procedure. In fact, I recall one woman who played Madonna's record "Like a Virgin" during the egg-retrieval process, bringing some levity to a very stressful situation.

If you are a man you may also find music or videos helpful to distract you from the stress of having to produce a semen sample, especially if you're under the intense pressure of the IVF procedure, when your partner's eggs have been harvested and they're waiting for your contribution to begin the fertilization process. Other useful distractions that clients have used while waiting for a procedure to begin include reading, doing crossword puzzles, knitting, and doing needlepoint.

Pain Medications

When you are dealing with the pain or discomfort of treatment it is important to remember that you don't have to be stoic and just tough it out. Dealing with infertility treatment is difficult enough without putting extra pressure on yourself to experience acute or prolonged pain. Indeed, medical staff are aware that some procedures can be uncomfortable and that some of the fertility medications are associated with painful side effects such as headaches. That's why many suggest the use of mild pain relievers to help ease your discomfort.

However, you may be reluctant to take any drugs. You've probably heard repeatedly how important it is for pregnant women to refrain from the use of medications or alcohol. You've also probably spent months or years trying to make your body as healthy as possible just in case you get pregnant. So, if you're like most women, you'll probably be reluctant to take any pain medication for fear that you might reduce your chances of a successful pregnancy or do harm to the fetus if the treatment in question is successful.

Know, however, that clinics would not offer pain medication if they felt that your taking it would reduce your chance of a successful pregnancy or cause harm to the fetus. If medication is offered, and you're concerned about your ability to cope with the discomfort, then it may be best to take it. If you're experiencing the side effects of superovulation medications, and you need some pain relief to be able to handle your job and your life, then check with your physician's office to find out what types of pain relievers they recommend.

Coping with Anxiety

As I've indicated throughout this chapter, medical fertility testing and treatments add to the anxiety you and your partner are already experiencing by being unable to produce a child. To a certain degree, this is inevitable, given the invasive nature of the investigations and interventions, and given the tremendous emotional and financial investment you have in the process. While it is impossible to eliminate this anxiety completely as long as you're going through treatment, it can be helpful to be familiar with the characteristic symptoms of anxiety, and some ways that can help you cope.

Some of the most common physical signs of heightened anxiety include difficulty sleeping, changes in appetite, dizziness, lower back pain, headaches, neck pain, nausea, shakiness, and shortness of breath. Psychological symptoms include inability to concentrate, forgetfulness, feeling fearful or panicky, loss of interest in activities you had previously enjoyed, and feeling easily annoyed and irritated. Anxiety can also be apparent in your relationships with others. You may find yourself being unusually short-tempered and hypersensitive with your partner or other significant people in your life. Things that you normally wouldn't care about may seem to be major issues, and you may find that you and your partner are fighting over really insignificant things.

While these symptoms are unpleasant, they are pretty normal, especially under the circumstances. In most situations in life, anxiety is an adaptive response. It alerts you to a threat and causes you to either flee the situation or take action to reduce the threat. This is commonly known as the "fight or flight" response. Once the threat is removed, the anxiety is reduced and you return to your normal state of functioning.

With fertility issues, however, the threat is usually ongoing. Until you achieve a viable pregnancy, the threat of childlessness persists. You can act to try to reduce this threat (the fight response) by pursuing treatment, but treatment is full of its own stresses and creates its own anxiety in addition to the anxiety you're already experiencing. Or you can try to flee (the flight response) by focusing on other things in your life and not addressing your infertility, but you're still faced with childlessness. So it's difficult to strike some balance, and it's difficult to handle ongoing anxiety.

It is unlikely that you're going to be able to completely eliminate your anxiety as long as you're involved in treatment. However, there are some things you can do to help *manage* your anxiety.

- Try to incorporate the progressive relaxation exercise discussed earlier in this chapter into your daily life, if only for five or ten minutes per day, while you're involved in treatment.

- Use self-hypnosis and visualizations to decrease your anxiety during stressful or painful procedures.

- To lessen some of the physical symptoms of anxiety, be sure that you eat right and that you exercise regularly, even if this means just walking.

- Try practicing yoga and meditation on a regular basis to reduce anxiety.

- Find an outlet for expressing your many fears and feelings about being infertile and having to go through fertility treatments. You may find support groups helpful, or you may have a trusted friend or family member who can listen to your struggles, without judging, and provide support.

- If you like to write, try keeping a journal. A journal can be a wonderful place to unload your feelings and it is always available to you, day and night.

- Play a musical instrument, take dance classes, or try your hand at art in order to express your feelings and lessen your anxiety.

- Challenge your negative thoughts and talk. Whenever you find yourself thinking or saying something negative, like "We'll never get pregnant; this is never going to work," say to yourself, "STOP! This isn't helpful." Then say something positive, such as, "If it's meant to be, it will happen," or "We're doing everything we can, and that's all we can expect of ourselves." Repeat these thought-stopping statements whenever you find yourself slipping into negative thinking or self-talk.

- Allow humor into your life; don't let the seriousness of infertility pervade every aspect of your day. Choose humorous movies to watch and lighthearted books to read. Let yourself laugh every now and then.

Coping with the Indignities of Testing and Treatment

The organs and body parts that are the primary focus of medical fertility investigations and treatment are the ones normally accorded the greatest degree of privacy. They are the ones that we make a point of keeping from public view and share only with those with whom we have an intimate relationship. It can be very embarrassing and humiliating to have these body parts repeatedly subjected to medical scrutiny.

If you are a man, your testicles will be examined and maybe even operated on. During the course of treatment, you'll be required to produce several semen samples so that your sperm can be tested or prepared for use during procedures. As Don, a forty-eight-year-old firefighter whose vasectomy reversal was unsuccessful, says:

You have no idea how hard it was to go into that little room carrying my brown paper bag containing the sterile sperm collection bottle. I just sat there for the longest time. There were erotic magazines and even some videos. But nothing helped. There was absolutely nothing erotic or sexy about being in this little room with a plastic bottle. How could anybody expect to get turned on in that kind of situation? And the longer I sat there, the more difficult it was. It was really tough. And, as if that wasn't bad enough, when I finally managed to produce a sample, I had to give it to the lab technician so she could assess the amount and quality of my sperm. If I had enough good-quality sperm I would pass. If I didn't I would fail—fail at being a man.

If you're a woman, you'll have your tubes, uterus, and vagina examined and reexamined. You'll likely be weighed. You may be injected with dye and drugs, scanned, and inseminated. Whether you're going through ovulation induction, inseminations, or IVF, you'll spend more time than you'd like with your feet in stirrups and your legs spread, a position that can feel very embarrassing and humiliating. After years of being told to cover up the most private parts of your body, you may feel shame at having your genitals repeatedly exposed to medical personnel, however supportive they may be in trying to help you become pregnant. Elaine, a thirty-two-year-old travel agent, explains it this way:

> Every time I turned around I was taking my clothes off and having someone stick a speculum or ultrasound probe into my vagina, or a catheter into my cervix. At first it was really difficult. I'd tense up and it would be very painful. Over time I found ways to relax so that it wasn't as uncomfortable . . . but I never got used to it. It was never easy.

There are no easy ways to cope with the invasiveness and indignities of medical testing and treatment. However, using progressive relaxation and controlled breathing techniques can help you to relax your body during these procedures, and practicing visualization can help you to cope with the feeling of violation. You can make a point of asking to be left alone when you're getting dressed or undressed. Insist on having a gown or sheet to cover yourself. Ask that the staff knock before entering the examination or procedure room. Ask to have the speculum warmed before it is inserted. Ask to be introduced to the medical specialist, before you take your clothes off and are lying down with your feet in stirrups. Ask to have your partner be present if you'd find this helpful.

When you have to provide a semen sample, try to make the appointment for a time in the day when you're more likely to find this easier. For some men, this might mean providing a sample first thing in the morning so they won't have to worry about it all day. For others, it may mean waiting until the end of the day, when there is less pressure to get back to work. Bring your own magazines or videos if you'd find these helpful. You may find it helpful to have your partner with you, rather than producing the sample alone. If you think producing a sample on demand at the clinic will be too difficult for you, ask whether you can produce the sample in a more comfortable setting, perhaps at a nearby hotel or, if you live close enough to the lab, in your own bedroom.

The most important thing to remember as you struggle to deal with these challenges is that you can exercise some control over the conditions of testing and treatment. So, decide what you need in order to make this process as comfortable as possible for yourself, and communicate this to the medical staff in a way that acknowledges your needs, while also being respectful of theirs. For example, if you're about to go through egg retrieval and haven't yet met the physician who will be doing this procedure, you can simply say, "I know everyone is probably very busy this morning, but I haven't had a chance to meet the doctor who'll be doing my retrieval. I'm pretty nervous, as you can imagine, so if she/he has a minute before we get started, it would really help me to have a chance to meet her/him and just say hello."

Coping with Anger

While you are going through medical testing and treatment you may well find yourself uncharacteristically angry and short-tempered. Little things that your partner says or does bug you. You're irritated with the people at work, and you've had it with your friends and family members who seem to talk about nothing but their kids. You're tired of waiting for tests and appointments—after all, you're a busy person too. And, if the receptionist at the clinic insists on publicly announcing why you're here one more time, you just might climb over the desk and deck her! Indeed, much of the anger you experience during this process may be directed at the medical staff who are treating you.

Needless to say, anger and frustration are very normal responses to the injustices of infertility, and to the stresses of medical testing and treatment. You have a lot riding on these people, who are supposed to be finding answers and solutions to your fertility problems, and time is marching on. Under these circumstances, it's hard to keep perspective and it usually doesn't take much to make you snap. This is especially the case if your test results have been misfiled, for example, or your physician inadvertently makes a mistake with your treatment protocol, which happened to Tracy, a thirty-four-year-old waitress:

> The thing that really got me angry was that the doctor got me mixed up with someone else. I had a laparoscopy and after the surgery he told my husband I had endometriosis. And then the next morning when the doctor came around to visit me, he

told me everything was fine! I said, "What about the endometriosis?" And when he looked in my chart he said, "No, you don't have endometriosis. Where did you get that idea?"

Jan, a thirty-eight-year-old court reporter, talks about similar problems in the management of her treatment.

The first time we went through IVF it didn't work. I didn't respond well to the drugs, so the cycle had to be canceled. When I met with the doctor, he said we could do it again, only next time they'd use a different combination of drugs. So we waited another six months to start our next cycle, and when we began they prescribed the same medications that I had the first time. I said, "Hey, wait a minute, I thought we weren't using these drugs again." My doctor looked at my chart and said, "Oh, sorry, you're right. I guess we forgot." Here we are spending thousands of dollars and running out of time, and they just say, "Sorry, we forgot."

It can be enormously frustrating to experience these kinds of mistakes, and if they happen, you have every right to be upset. However, remember that the people who are trying to help you are only human. They can, and sometimes do, make mistakes. This is all the more reason for you to become an expert on your own case, to help ensure that something important doesn't get missed or overlooked.

Fear and Anger

When people get angry, a lot of the time it's because they're scared. Anger is usually an easier emotion to express and experience than fear, especially for men. So if you find that you're angry all the time, it can be helpful to ask yourself what you're afraid of. Perhaps you're afraid that you'll find out your sperm or eggs aren't viable. Perhaps you're afraid that your tubes are irreparably damaged, or that your uterus won't be able to carry a pregnancy. Perhaps you're afraid that, after all of the tests and treatment—all of the effort, discomfort, and expense—the doctors still won't be able to tell you why you're unable to get pregnant. Perhaps you're afraid that your worst fears will come true and your childlessness will be permanent.

Your Worst Fears: Preparing for Bad News

The possibility of bad news always hangs over your heads when you're going through medical testing and treatment. While you want to remain optimistic and are hopeful that medical science will be able to identify the problem and find a workable solution, you are also always aware and fearful of the fact that they may not. Every time you take a new test or undergo a treatment cycle, you are aware of the fact that the news might not be good. On the one hand, you fear that your doctors will find that something's wrong. On the other hand, you fear that they won't and you won't be any further ahead after all your efforts.

It's never easy to prepare for bad news, even if you know at some level that it's coming. You may have had some heavy spotting since your insemination or embryo transfer and have a pretty good suspicion that treatment didn't work, but it's still hard to take when you hear that your blood test came back negative. You may know that your sperm count isn't great, but it can still be pretty devastating to find out that, even with all the new technology, you can't make a baby.

Nevertheless, there are still a few things you can do to make it easier on yourselves.

1. Try to maintain an attitude of cautious optimism discussed at the beginning of this chapter. It will be easier for you to hear bad news, and to cope with it, if you haven't set yourself up to believe that medical science can definitely identify and fix the problem. Absolutist thinking won't serve you well in this type of situation.

2. Try not to go alone to medical appointments. Have your partner with you when discussing test results or treatment options with your health-care provider. If your partner isn't available, take someone else. It can be very helpful to have emotional and physical support—someone to drive you home and feed you chicken soup. If you have to call the clinic to find out the results of a test and you think you'll get bad news, have your partner call instead if you think you won't be able to handle it. It can sometimes be easier if he or she is the one to break the news to you, rather than a nurse or receptionist.

3. Try to book medical consultations or tests for a time when you don't have to go to work immediately. It can be extremely difficult to conduct business when you've just been told that they can't find a heart beat on the ultrasound and that you will probably miscarry, or that none of your embryos fertilized, or that they weren't able to get the sperm they needed from your partner's testicles. No one would expect you to function normally if you'd just been told your child had died, and that's pretty much what is happening when you get this kind of bad news. The child you'd hoped for and perhaps even prayed for may never be, and it's like a death. So don't expect too much of yourself.

4. If you get bad news, take some time to let it sink in. Avoid the tendency to immediately begin another treatment cycle or another treatment option. It can indeed be comforting to hear your physician saying that there are options available. So if it's helpful, get the information and take it home with you. Then take a few days, or even a few weeks or months, before making any decisions. None of us make our best decisions when we're in crisis, so if you want to make decisions you can live with, give yourself a bit of time after getting bad news to regroup and recover, and perhaps to grieve.

Look Before You Leap

Even if you haven't received bad news, it is still beneficial to take a bit of time between treatments to gather some information on your options and the probabilities of success. It is also important for each of you to take your "emotional temperature." What this means is that you examine your feelings. If one of you is still very distressed about your diagnosis and having some difficulty thinking about treatment options, or if either of you are uncomfortable with the option being recommended by your physician, you should probably take some time before making a decision. The words of Anne, a thirty-seven-year-old teacher, show how hard it can be to disengage from the process and think over your options:

A lot of the time that you're going through treatment, you're just running on automatic pilot so that you don't even realize what you're doing or you don't even give it a lot of thought because if you do, you're afraid it just might drive you over the edge. During treatment it's like there's a certain length of

*time that exists and that's the time until your next
appointment or your next treatment cycle. It's like you're on a
ride and don't get off the ride until it's over. And only then
do you realize that somewhere along the way you lost your
perspective, and maybe even yourself.*

Forty-one-year-old David, a steelworker, describes it as a
vicious cycle:

*You're doing things that you probably would never ever
consider if you were in your right mind . . . but you're not
in your right mind. That's the problem. You're hooked into a
cycle—a vicious cycle. And just when you think you're ready
to give up, you hear about someone who kept on trying and
finally got pregnant, and you think, "That could be us!" So
you stay hooked into treatment, even when your chances aren't
great. After all, nobody would bet their life savings in Vegas
with odds of only 15 or 20 percent, but it's different when it
comes to having a baby.*

The decisions you're making now can affect the rest of your life.
So take your time to consider the range of options, and read about
and consider the pros and cons—medical, legal, social, and ethical—of your various options, especially if you're thinking about moving to a third-party reproductive option. I've worked with couples
who moved to this type of option before one of them was ready, as
with the example of Susan and Ted in chapter 2. They faced some
difficult emotional work after they finally achieved a pregnancy,
because the partner who was not genetically involved in creating the
child had difficulty accepting the pregnancy. This work is much easier to do *before*, rather than after, a pregnancy begins. Otherwise,
what should be a joyous event can become a serious crisis.

Will This Never End?: Coping with Failed Treatment

When you go through infertility a sense of failure seems to be your
common companion. You constantly encounter the monthly reminders that you're not yet pregnant. Thirty-five-year-old Sarah refers to it
as the monthly cycle of dashed hopes:

*Every month it's the same story. We go through the hope and
despair. For the first two weeks of my cycle we're hopeful, and*

for the next two we're despairing. The months just keep on ticking by with no end in sight.

This cycle becomes even more intense when you're going through fertility investigations and treatments. When you begin a treatment cycle, you're filled with hope, or cautious optimism, that this time it's going to work. You do everything you can to make sure you're giving treatment your best shot. And yet, despite your best efforts, you don't get pregnant. Or if you do, maybe you end up miscarrying a few weeks later. After three failed IVF cycles, thirty-six-year-old interior designer Cheryl describes the despair that follows a failed treatment cycle:

> *The odds they quote are pretty optimistic . . . like you have a 20 or 25 percent chance of getting pregnant. So at the beginning it's always this upbeat sort of thing. You start the cycle thinking, yeah, I'm gonna be in that 20 percent, this time it's gonna work, this time it's our turn. And then it doesn't happen and you're back in the depths of despair.*

It's hard not to blame yourself or your partner. It's difficult not to blame your body for not functioning right. It's hard not to think that somehow you did something wrong—that somehow it's your fault, or your partner's fault, that you're not pregnant. Unfortunately, the medical language doesn't help either. Although medical professionals are more sensitive in their use of diagnostic language than in the past, some of their words can have a negative connotation. When you're told that your eggs or sperm are "inadequate" or of "poor quality," your ovaries aren't "responsive," your mucus is "hostile," or your cervix is "incompetent" or "forbidding," it's pretty difficult not to feel that this is your personal failure.

To help you cope and maintain some sense of your own efficacy as a man or a woman, it is *critical* that you understand that it is medical science and medical treatment that have failed, not you! You need to reject any tendency to assume that if treatment is successful, your physicians were the ones who got you pregnant, but if treatment isn't successful that it's your fault. You need to reject blaming and negative language; refuse to allow it to define you or your body.

You also need to reframe the whole notion of failure. Is it fair to consider yourself a failure because you were unfortunate enough to have undescended testicles or a groin injury when you were a child? Is it fair to consider yourself a failure because your pituitary gland isn't producing the right hormones in the right quantities, or your tubes are scarred, or you have endometriosis, or the lining of your uterus isn't as thick as it needs to be to maintain a pregnancy?

No. It's not fair, and it's not your fault. Simply put, life is not fair. You've been dealt a bad hand and you're doing your best to play it. You're putting time and energy and money into trying to find answers, and you're taking the risk to pursue solutions. Medical science is amazing, but it is still limited in what it can provide. If you try what science has to offer, and it doesn't work, it is the limitations of science that you're bumping up against, not your own limitations. *You didn't cause your infertility and you can't cure it. But you can try, within the limits of your resources, to overcome it—that's all you can do.*

5

We're in This Together: Keeping Your Relationship Alive

Infertility challenges everything . . . your beliefs about yourself, about what's important in life, about marriage, about what is fair and just, about God. Being infertile makes you question the purpose of marriage and of life . . . Nothing is left unaffected by this experience . . . it changes you, subtly but profoundly. I think that the biggest thing that we've had to work through as a couple and me as a person is just learning to live with it . . . because being infertile changes everything.

As is so eloquently stated by Tom, the thirty-nine-year-old man speaking above, the experience of being unable to produce a child, and the often prolonged pursuit of answers and solutions to this problem, inevitably touches on all aspects of your lives together. The experience affects the way you see yourself and your partner, and it has an effect on your relationship. Like other difficult and challenging life experiences, going through infertility together can ultimately strengthen your relationship with your partner. However, while you're going through it, you may find that it places stresses on your marriage unlike any you've experienced. It will inevitably be a rocky road, but how you cope with these stresses together, and how you communicate with each other about your feelings, fears, concerns, and needs, will affect whether infertility takes a toll on your relationship or brings you closer together as a couple.

The issues discussed below are the ones most commonly encountered by infertile couples, especially when they're going through medical fertility testing and treatments. To varying degrees they will probably reflect your experiences as well. The suggestions provided in this chapter should help to keep you more connected to, and appreciative of, the person with whom you'd like to create a child—your partner.

"Maybe You Should Find Someone Else": Being the Infertile Partner

How you and your partner react to infertility, and how you feel about yourself and your relationship, will likely have a lot to do with which one of you is identified as having the fertility problem. As a couple going through infertility, you will both experience feelings of loss about the child you may not be able to create together. However, if you are the partner who is diagnosed with the physical impairment you will most likely also experience a range of other difficult emotions.

You may feel that you are physically defective, that your body has failed you. Infertility can have a very negative effect on your body image, making it difficult to feel comfortable sharing your body with your partner. The invasiveness of the medical examinations and procedures will likely only add to these feelings. That's why it's necessary to continue to take care of yourself, emotionally and physically. *Try to frame infertility, not your body, as the problem.* Remember that your identity consists of a great deal more than the quality of your sperm or eggs, or the condition of your tubes or uterus.

You may believe that your infertility is somehow your fault. You feel guilty for not trying to become pregnant earlier or not seeking medical help sooner. Guilt usually isn't rational, making it difficult to control. Even if you had initiated efforts to have children when you were younger, your sperm count would not necessarily have been any higher, or the quality of your eggs necessarily any better. Women can go into premature ovarian failure in their twenties, and some men with poor sperm quality or an obstruction in the sperm ducts have the problem from puberty. As thirty-six-year-old Ian describes below, guilt may lead you to believe that you owe it to your partner to do whatever is necessary, whatever it takes to try to have a child:

> *How could I possibly tell her I wouldn't participate in any more treatment or that I wasn't willing to consider donor sperm or adoption. After all, it was my fault that we were going through all this . . . it was my fault that I wasn't able to fulfill my role and give her a baby. Whatever she wanted, it had to be okay with me, even if what she wanted was a different partner who could give her a baby.*

The problem with this kind of thinking is that you may end up agreeing to try a treatment or parenting option that you really aren't comfortable with and can't live with in the long run. So if you find yourself agreeing to pursue an option you didn't think you'd ever be willing to consider, then you need to seriously ask yourself why you're agreeing to this. If your answer is that you feel guilty or you feel you owe it to your partner because it's your fault she or he can't have a child, then you need to talk to your partner about your feelings and take the time to rethink your decision. You may eventually come to the same conclusion, but if you pursue a treatment or parenting option, you need to be sure that it's an option you feel committed to and truly can live with—not something you're doing out of guilt.

Communicating your feelings to your partner if you're the one with the identified fertility problem is often easier said than done because it means you first have to acknowledge these feelings to yourself. So if one of you becomes reluctant to talk with the other about your infertility, it may be because you're afraid of facing these very painful feelings. Ed, a forty-three-year-old minister diagnosed with obstructive azoospermia, puts it this way:

> *I did not want to seriously examine my feelings because I did not want to face my pain, sorrow, disappointment, and inadequacy . . . and I did not want to hear my wife's feelings of pain and anger about my infertility . . . a lot of it was not having the ability to honestly say what I was feeling.*

If you do allow yourself to acknowledge your feelings, you will most likely experience tremendous sadness and grief, possibly unlike any you've experienced before. Jim, a thirty-four-year-old computer analyst, describes it this way:

> *It was more grief than I had with the loss of my grandfather . . . whom I loved more than anyone when I was a child. It*

*was just grief—physical, emotional grief, that I had lost this
gift, this ability—fertility. I couldn't cope with the fact that I
would never see, never have a child, a biological child who
would have some of my characteristics. It felt like such a
tragedy.*

Because fertility is so closely tied to our notions of masculinity
and femininity it's also pretty common to feel that you are less of a
man or woman because you can't produce a child. Like Sam, a thirty-
year-old insurance adjuster whose sperm count deteriorated following radiation treatments for testicular cancer, you may also feel inadequate as a lover, and as a partner, because you feel you're denying
your spouse something that is very important to both of you.

*A man should be able to have children and be able to give his
wife children. So it was simple: because I couldn't, I wasn't a
real man . . . simple, straightforward. That's why I felt an
attack on my maleness. It all comes down to one
word—inadequate. I felt totally and completely inadequate, as
a man and as a husband.*

Like thirty-four-year-old Martha, the infertile woman speaking
in the following quote, your feelings of inadequacy and guilt may
lead you to feel that your partner should find someone else, with
whom he or she can have a child:

*It's such an emotional roller coaster and you have such a wide
range of emotions. You feel like you're not normal because if
you're a woman you should be able to reproduce. You feel like
telling your partner, "Why don't you just go and have a baby
with someone else and just come back later. Just leave the
relationship, leave me, you don't deserve this, you deserve
better than what I have to offer."*

You may find yourself looking outside your relationship to confirm that you're still attractive, adequate, and desirable. Or, you may
find that you're angry about everything your partner says or does,
when in fact what you're really angry at is the injustice of your
infertility.

In order to avoid serious long-term damage to your relationship, you must find a way to communicate your feelings to your
partner. You need to let your partner know that you're not rejecting
him or her—that you don't want the relationship to end. You need to
let your partner know that your behaviors are based on your feelings
of inadequacy and guilt. These aren't always easy things to admit or

express, so you might consider writing your thoughts and feelings in a letter to your partner, as Doug, a thirty-eight–year-old musician, did:

> *With a lump in my throat I wrote that I felt unmanly, inadequate, and powerless when I compared myself to other men who have children. I also explained that I felt inadequate sometimes when my performance as a sexual partner wasn't perfect . . . and I told her I'd give her the freedom to find a more worthy, manly husband who could give her the children she wanted and deserved.*

Open and honest communication about issues that touch on your sense of inadequacy as a woman or man, and on your feelings of sexual inadequacy, can be very difficult. To address these issues requires real trust in your partner and a belief that she or he will not reject you. However, expressing your painful feelings is most often worth the risk. You may well find that your partner, the person who loves you enough to want to have a child with you, is aware of your pain and is supportive of you in your struggles. As twenty-nine-year-old Cynthia found out, it can be tremendously reassuring to know that your partner loves you for who you are as a person and as a partner, not just for your ability to reproduce:

> *One of the very critical things that he does in terms of support for me is to continually assure me that our marriage is complete, even without children and that he loves me all the same, whether I can produce a child or not . . . and that makes all the difference to me. I can cope with all the pain and loss knowing that my marriage is on solid ground.*

"But I Don't Want Anyone Else": Being the Fertile Partner

In some ways it is easier to cope with infertility if you are the partner who is given the clean bill of health. However, this role is not without its difficulties. Initially, when you are told that your test results don't show any problems, you will likely feel relief. You are still a member of an infertile couple, but at least everything is okay on your end.

If you are a woman, the fact that the fertility problem is related to your partner's physiology and not yours may well surprise you.

Fertility is often considered a woman's issue and most women assume when there is a problem getting pregnant, that it's because something is wrong with them. Even in cases where there has been some indication of a male factor problem at the outset, perhaps due to undescended testicles, an early groin injury, or previous chemotherapy and radiation, most women still assume that there must be something wrong with their bodies because they aren't getting pregnant. And their partners share this assumption. Lyle, a thirty-four year old police officer who was diagnosed as having no sperm, put it this way:

> I just assumed that it obviously wasn't my problem, it had to be hers. Infertility is not a male problem, it's a female problem. The woman can't have the baby. Not the man, it's the woman. That's why I was so shocked when they said it was my sperm. I just thought it would be my wife's problem, and so did she. We were both really surprised.

Interestingly, if you're like many women, you may continue to assume that you are also infertile even after all your tests indicate otherwise and your partner has been identified with a male factor problem. Other people will likely also assume that you are the infertile partner. You may even find yourself confirming these assumptions, as a way to avoid having to offer explanations, and as a way to protect your male partner's feelings. Initially this approach may work for both of you, but over time it can become a problem to maintain the illusion that the problem is yours and that you are responsible for not producing the grandchildren that your parents or your partner's parents desperately want. You may eventually find yourself getting resentful at having to take the blame for a problem in your partner's physiology, not yours.

Another common reaction to your partner's infertility is anger. Anger is a frightening emotion in most relationships, one that many people, especially women, have difficulty dealing effectively with. But it is an understandable reaction to being denied something as important in life as the chance to produce a child. Thirty-two-year-old Christine describes her reaction to a similar husband's diagnosis of a low sperm count.

> I hated to admit that I felt that way, but I was really angry. After all, I was the fertile one, and yet if we were going to have any chance at all of having our own child I was going to have to take all the drugs, and go through all the painful procedures, and disrupt my life for weeks on end. All because

his sperm were lousy. It just wasn't fair. It was his fault that
we weren't getting pregnant, but I had to put my body
through all that crap. And do you know what's really ironic?
One of the reasons I was attracted to him in the first place
was that he was so masculine . . . with his big shoulders and
chest, and his square jaw. I thought he was a real specimen of
a macho guy. And now look—his sperm are practically
useless!

It is normal to feel this way when you first learn that your partner is unable to produce a child, but these feelings usually subside over time. Although your anger is a legitimate emotion it often serves to cover up deeper feelings of loss and grief. So if you find yourself feeling angry about your partner's fertility problem, it may be helpful for you to find some healthy outlets for your feelings, perhaps through journaling, art, or some intense physical activity (e.g., sports, exercise, dance). These outlets would be less destructive than to verbally attack your partner, who is no doubt already feeling bad enough about his or her infertility. Rather than letting your anger fester or come out in unhealthy ways, talk about your feelings with your partner, focusing on your anger at the injustice of infertility, rather than at your partner's fertility problem. Also, try to get in touch with, and express, the feelings that are underneath your anger. You may find that your feelings of loss, grief, and sadness are easier to share with your partner than you had expected, because she or he is experiencing these as well.

As the partner with the clean bill of health—the fertile partner—you may also feel some guilt because you're physically okay and your partner is not. This is not unlike survivor guilt, felt by people who have lived through an accident or tragedy in which others did not survive. In this case, you've escaped the infertility bullet, but your partner has not. As a consequence, you may find yourself walking on eggshells, not certain about what to say to help him or her cope or feel better, perhaps even afraid to discuss other treatment or parenting options for fear that you'll only add to his or her feelings of inadequacy. The issue of infertility is a bit like an elephant in a living room: it takes up a lot of space in your lives and relationship, but you tiptoe around the issue for fear of getting an angry reaction from your partner or causing him or her more pain.

While this kind of reaction is understandable and normal, it also can be problematic, especially if you're up against some very real time restrictions. Like thirty-nine-year-old Lucy, you may find yourself getting frustrated and resentful because you feel that, in your efforts to be sensitive to your partner's feelings, you may be giving up your only chance to become a parent. Ultimately neither of you wins with this kind of approach.

> *It was so incredibly frustrating. When we found out about my husband's sperm problem I knew he was devastated. We both were. So we decided to just let it go for a while. I was already thirty-seven and I knew the clock was ticking, but I didn't feel like I could push him. And every time I even raised the issue of treatment, he'd get upset and we'd get into a terrible fight. It went on like that for two years. Two years! Finally, I couldn't take it any more. Time was running out, and if we didn't do something soon I'd knew I'd never get pregnant. It became a crisis and we had to get some help—we just couldn't seem to tackle this one on our own. But we got there, eventually. A year or two later than I'd have liked, but we got there.*

By all means give yourselves some time after a diagnosis to let the reality of the situation sink in. Don't automatically begin pursuing a treatment or parenting option that you haven't already talked about and agreed to before. But don't let the issue go unaddressed for too long. The feelings you both have, although not necessarily entirely the same, need to be acknowledged and expressed—verbally or in writing. And they need to be shared. If you find that you can't do this on your own, get some counseling, because if you end up childless in the long run because one of you refused to seriously consider the available options, the seeds of resentment may eventually put your marriage at risk. So, however painful, address your feelings—verbally or in writing—together or with a counselor. Only then will you both be able to move forward in your decision making.

"It's Our Problem": Reframing Infertility as a Couple's Issue

When one of you is identified as having a fertility impairment, it is natural to see that partner as the source of the problem. The reality, however, is that the inability to produce a child together is not an individual problem, it is a *couple's problem*. The child you dream of and want to create would share your genetic histories, and have your partner's blue eyes or red hair or sense of humor. It was because you care deeply about your partner that you decided she or he was the person you wanted to parent with, not someone else. And although it is sometimes easy to lose sight of this reality, try to remember that it is your *mutual loss* that you are not able to produce a child together.

Accordingly, it is really important that you treat infertility not as your partner's problem or your problem but as your mutual problem—something that you need to tackle together. From your initial decision to start trying to have a family to your choices about which tests, treatments, and which parenting options to pursue, you need to walk this road together. Your decisions need to be joint decisions. Whenever possible, attend your medical appointments together, so that you can share the responsibility for keeping these appointments and getting information about your options.

Shared decision making and participation in treatment is especially important if you are considering a third-party reproductive option, such as using donor sperm or eggs. For example, sometimes men are uncomfortable looking through sperm donor profiles and want to defer the decision making to their wives. To protect their partners from having to be confronted with their infertility, women sometimes agree to take on this responsibility. However, if a man isn't comfortable selecting the donor who will provide 50 percent of the genetic material of the child, how comfortable will he be with the child when she or he is born? Not being willing to participate in the donor selection process is often an indication that a man hasn't reconciled himself to his infertility. It may indicate that he is not comfortable with the fact that his wife will be inseminated with the sperm of another man; he may even feel that this is a bit like infidelity. In the woman's attempt to protect her partner from having to confront his infertility by not insisting that he participate in the donor selection process, she may actually be reinforcing the insignificance of his contribution to the creation of the child. And when treatment begins, if the man stays in his office, in the parking lot, or in the waiting room while the woman is going through donor insemination, he is likely to feel even less involved in the creation of his child.

The same advice applies to the adoption process. If you decide to apply for adoption, you both need to participate in this effort. Not only will it reinforce your mutual commitment to the option, as thirty-six-year-old Lydia describes below it will also help you to feel that as a couple you're capable of making your goal of parenthood a reality.

> We were doing something together, which felt great . . . and in the end, if we were going to have a child out of the whole process that would be wonderful, but even if we weren't, just

*our being together in this was worth it. It really was.
Through this process of infertility we've learned who our
support people are . . . and that's each other. A child will just
be the icing on the cake.*

So, whenever possible, make every effort to work together on considering and pursuing treatment and parenting options, and to frame your struggles as a mutual effort to cope with the real problem—childlessness. In particular, be aware of the language you use related to your infertility. Be careful to use inclusive language such as "our infertility," rather than "your infertility," and "our problem," rather than "my problem." If you end up using a third-party option to create your family, be very careful to refer to the child you are creating together as "our child," rather than "my child" or "your child." Also, try not to use words like "real" or "natural" parent in reference to the donor who provides the sperm or eggs. The reality is that, no matter where the sperm or eggs come from, you and your partner are both making an emotional commitment and contribution to the creation and raising of your child, and that makes you the "real" and "natural" parents.

Gender Differences in Response to Infertility

The fact that you are in this together, however, doesn't mean that you will experience infertility and childlessness in the same way. It also doesn't mean that you'll respond to your inability to have a family in a similar manner, or on a similar time schedule. There are many differences in the way men and women respond to infertility, and these differences can make communication and decision making more difficult.

For example, women frequently react with more overt emotion to their inability to produce a child. Infertile women usually experience more anxiety and depression than their infertile partners. Women are usually much more sensitive to the comments of other people regarding their childless status. If you are a woman going through treatment you may also find yourself experiencing physical and psychological symptoms in response to your distress, including headaches, back and neck pain, difficulties concentrating, and memory loss. Whether or not you are the partner identified with the physical problem, your self-esteem will likely suffer as a consequence of dealing with infertility and medical treatment. The longer you have to continue without answers or solutions to your infertility, the greater your distress is likely to be. Your partner, on the other hand, will likely experience and express his feelings about not being able to have a child a bit differently.

If you're a man you may be distressed at being unable to produce a child, but you are more likely to be upset by your partner's obvious distress and your inability to fix the situation. While you won't necessarily be able to relate to her distress at not being able to experience pregnancy and childbirth, you will likely appreciate that this is something important to many women and regret that your partner may never have the chance to experience it. You may not have the same investment in trying to have a child as your partner does, and you may find yourself going along with the treatment options that your partner wants to pursue with a lower level of commitment to the process than she seems to have. You may initially cope with the whole thing by keeping yourself busy with other things and by avoiding talking about your infertility. Thirty-seven-year-old Nathan, an officer in the army, describes his reluctance to address the pain of his infertility in these words:

> If my wife was sobbing at night on one side of the bed, I
> would just turn over and not be of any sort of comfort . . . I
> couldn't really listen to her . . . to what she was
> communicating and the feelings of emptiness . . . the feelings
> of being alone, of feeling hurt. My reaction was to be very
> silent, withdrawing, not wanting to talk about it because I
> knew I couldn't fix it, and it killed me to think I couldn't
> stop her pain.

Or your approach may be to try to stay positive and optimistic. But eventually, like forty-three-year-old Barry, a year or two after your partner has been continuously immersed in pain and grief, you may start to experience some of the same symptoms of depression and feelings of loss:

> I was quite a ways behind her in terms of the whole emotional
> impact. She would be grieving about it and be depressed and
> I'd say "Ah, come on, cheer up, you know, relax, get a grip."
> That kind of thing. About a year or so after that I started
> getting a little more depressed, down on life. Once that started
> happening I'd tell her and she was great—really helpful,
> because she'd gone through it already and knew only too well
> how I was feeling.

These types of gender differences in response to infertility are common and normal. As discussed in chapters 2 and 3, women's bodies are the primary focus of medical testing and treatment. This fact alone makes it more likely that the female partner will find the experience of medical treatment more distressing. Adding fertility medications to an already stressful situation increases the likelihood that women will experience fairly intense mood swings, contributing further to their distress. Women are also more connected to their fertility, and infertility, than men—the failure to conceive plays itself out in the woman's body every month. It makes sense, then, that childlessness would initially be experienced more intensely by a woman than it would be by her partner.

It is also important to realize that in our society, as in most societies throughout the world, women and the social worlds they inhabit are more defined by motherhood than men and their social worlds are. For example, as thirty-two-year-old Greg, a construction worker, comments below, if a man becomes a father his work life and his friendships with other men don't tend to change a great deal:

> It's funny, but even though my closest buddy became a dad this year, things really haven't changed much. We still play hockey every Friday night and get together for a beer or coffee after work a few times a week. We might make jokes now about how, when he gets home, he's handed a squawking baby with a dirty diaper while his wife, who really needs a break, heads for the gym . . . but overall things aren't really different.

For many women, however, their relationships with other women change considerably when they become mothers. Between their jobs and taking care of their kids, they don't have as much time for their childless friends. So, in addition to their childlessness, infertile women also have to cope with the pain of being excluded from the lives of their friends and family members who've made the transition to motherhood.

Differences in the ways you and your partner respond to being infertile also stem from the ways men and women are normally taught to respond to life situations. Women characteristically express more emotion than men. Women vent—men fix. Women talk—men watch TV, play sports, or bury themselves in work. These differences often lead to painful misunderstandings. A woman might start to believe that her husband doesn't care as much as she does about having a baby. A man might think that his wife cares more about having a baby than she does about him.

It is these assumptions that can get you into trouble in your marriage as you try to cope, together, with your infertility. That's why communication is so important. That's also why communicating effectively about infertility isn't always easy.

Communicating Effectively about Infertility

Given these very real gender differences in the experience of infertility and medical testing, and the sensitivity of the person in the relationship with the fertility problem, it wouldn't be surprising if you and your partner had some difficulty communicating effectively when it comes to this important issue. Communication problems are very common in any relationship during stressful situations, and dealing with infertility on an ongoing basis certainly qualifies as a very stressful experience. In addition, even though your goal of producing a child together may be the same, the stresses for you and your partner, and your investment in the outcome, are likely to be different. Even if your investment in becoming parents is the same, you probably won't experience the same feelings on the same schedule. This makes hearing and understanding each other more difficult, and more important.

In chapter 3 I talked about ways you can address and work through differences with your partner when you are having difficulty agreeing on a course of action to pursue. Focusing on infertility and childlessness (not your partner) as the enemy, being clear about your own needs, being respectful of your partner's feelings, and communicating directly are all useful techniques for surviving infertility together. The suggestions below may also help you understand your own perspective and needs as well as those of your partner, as you attempt to deal with your feelings about, and reactions to, infertility. While these suggestions can help you communicate more effectively, as forty-year-old Sandra says below, the most critical thing to remember is that *you are both in this together and your partner is your greatest ally in your struggles to have a family.*

> *It was a very difficult road. At times I felt like we were going*
> *in completely different directions . . . that we wanted*
> *completely different things. We had some incredible battles,*
> *and some cold wars that lasted for days—days we couldn't*
> *even speak to each other. At times I even thought about*

leaving the marriage. If he didn't want kids as bad as I did, then maybe we didn't have the same values after all. Maybe we really wanted different things in life. But we worked it through—we hung in there together, and it sure wasn't easy. But the fact that we were able to work out an issue this important, and this emotionally loaded, is something we can rely on for the rest of our lives.

Put Boundaries around Your Fertility Discussions

Over time, infertility can take up an enormous amount of space in your relationship. You may find that having kids, not having kids, and fertility treatments are all you seem to talk about. Being infertile can be an overwhelming experience. Talking about it constantly can be overwhelming too. It can take over your life. So you need to put some boundaries around your discussions about infertility, parenthood, and your treatment options, deciding when, where, how long, and how often you will talk about these issues.

You may decide to limit your discussions about infertility to a half hour each day, especially during treatment cycles. Or you may agree to put time aside to check in with each other during weekends, when there are fewer demands on your time and energy. Sort out what's workable for both of you, and try to stay within these agreed upon boundaries.

Also, pick a neutral place to have your discussions. Try not to have these conversations when you're in bed together. Infertility already takes a toll on your sexual spontaneity, and talking about it in bed only strengthens the connection between intimacy and failure. Dinner is also not usually the best time, whether you're out together or at home, because discussing infertility often brings up a lot of distressing emotions.

If you put some clear boundaries in place, you'll probably find that you accomplish more together when you do discuss your infertility. You'll probably make better decisions and deepen your understanding of your feelings and your partner's feelings about your situation. You may find that your partner is more willing to participate in these discussions if they are time-limited. Also by not allowing infertility to take up so much space in your life, you will ensure that there is some room in your lives to nurture some of the more pleasant and enjoyable aspects of your relationship.

Check Out Your Assumptions

One of the things that gets couples into a lot of trouble and makes communication more strained is when one partner interprets the other person's behavior in a negative or inaccurate way. For example, if you are a woman you will likely want to talk about your infertility and express the full range of your feelings of frustration, anger, sadness, loss, and grief. You may feel a need to vent, and in fact you may find that it helps to cry and scream a little. However, your partner may find it upsetting to see you so distressed, especially when he can't do anything to fix the problem. He may interpret your insistence on focusing so much on your infertility and pursuing endless treatment options to mean that you want to have a child at any cost—even at the expense of your relationship.

If you're a man you may avoid talking about infertility—after all, every time you do, your partner probably gets very upset and you can't do or say anything to make her feel better. She keeps talking about treatment options and seems obsessed with finding a solution to the problem, *at any cost*, or so it appears to you. So you suggest that maybe it's time for you to move on. Your partner may interpret your behavior to mean that you aren't as invested in having a child, aren't as committed to treatment, and aren't as bothered by your inability to have a child as she is. Neither of your assumptions may be accurate, and yet these can drive a wedge between you, cutting you off from your greatest source of support—each other.

So, an important rule for communicating effectively, is don't make assumptions. Rather than assuming that your partner feels a particular way, *ask your partner how he or she feels!* For example, if you say, "I know you don't care as much about having a child as I do," or "Not being able to have kids just isn't as big a deal for you as it is for me," you're making assumptions about how your partner feels and not giving him or her the opportunity to express themselves. Instead, you could say something like, "Until we got into this situation I never realized how important being a parent was to me. What's it been like for you?" If you reframe your statements as questions, while taking ownership of your own feelings and asking your partner about theirs, you stand a much better chance of getting an accurate understanding of what's really going on for your partner, and for yourself.

Learn What Infertility Means to Each of You

Being unable to produce a child means different things to different people. So does the experience of going through medical fertility testing and treatment. It is important, therefore, not to assume that infertility means the same thing to your partner as it does to you. The intensity of your reaction to infertility may differ depending on what it means to you, and these meanings will influence your feelings about yourself and your partner, and the treatment and parenting decisions you make. It is critical, then, that you talk to your partner candidly about what being unable to have a child means to you, both as an individual, and as a member of an infertile couple. Thirty-year-old Donna, a flight attendant who was diagnosed with premature ovarian failure, describes the inability to experience pregnancy and childbirth this way:

You know, for a woman it's twofold. One is to never have the opportunity to be a biological mother. Two is to never carry a child inside of you and feel what it's like to nurture another life in that way. To feel the awesome power of pushing a child into this world and hearing its first cries and knowing that you gave that child life. For the man it's really only the one thing—it's just not being a biological father, right? But for a woman it's two experiences in a lifetime that you lose—it's two huge losses, not just one.

It is also important to try to differentiate between what it means to each of you to be *infertile*, and what it means to be *childless*. Although very connected to each other, these two issues are not the same. By allowing yourselves to explore and discuss the different meanings that being able to produce a child and being able to parent a child hold for you, you may find that you are able to sort through your treatment and parenting options with greater clarity and understanding.

Say What You Mean and Mean What You Say

Because of the intense emotions that get stirred up when you can't produce a child and the tremendous stress of prolonged medical testing and treatment, it is not uncommon for your feelings of anger, depression, frustration, and grief to bleed into other parts of your relationship. This is especially the case when you're having difficulty talking openly about infertility, or when you're deadlocked over a particular treatment or parenting option. Suddenly you and your partner may find yourselves bickering with each other and blowing up over the most insignificant things. He leaves a wet towel or underwear on the bathroom floor and you go ballistic. She forgets to pick up the laundry on the way home from work and you lose it. It's the time of the month when you're ovulating and you find yourself picking a fight just before you go to bed, or one of you decides to go out for a few drinks after work instead of coming home.

Infertility stress can challenge your relationship in a way that's unlike most other things you'll experience together in your marriage. However, when your anxiety and frustration about your situation or about your partner's behavior start to play themselves out covertly, rather than overtly, this can cause even more distress and damage. This type of emotional guerrilla warfare is highly toxic and can erode the foundation upon which your relationship is built—a foundation of love, trust, and mutual respect.

When you find yourself irritated by all of the little things your partner is or is not doing, or when you find yourself focusing exclusively on the negative aspects of your relationship, stop and ask yourself what you're really upset about. Look a bit deeper at the source of your frustration or distress. When you've identified what's really bothering you, discuss this openly and honestly with your partner. Be clear, be specific, and be prepared to listen to his or her perspective as well, even if it isn't the same as yours. Thirty-six-year-old Joanne explains below how she and her forty-eight-year-old partner, Tim, have found a way to address their feelings about their infertility and the various options available to them:

> We've gotten much better at talking about what's happening
> for each of us and not letting the anger and hurt and negative
> self-talk build to a frenzy. We started a weekly ritual of sitting
> by the fire and having a glass of wine, or sometimes even a
> bottle of wine, and we just talk about it. Where are we now
> and what are we doing? How do we feel about it? Do we
> really want to do this? We ask each other how we're feeling,
> and we do our best not to get defensive. We keep it really
> open, because we both have a right to our feelings about this.
> That's what we do. We talk openly and honestly and try not
> to be defensive. So we both feel heard and we both feel
> understood, even if we don't always agree. I guess we've really

learned how to communicate through all of this. It's been our salvation through the toughest times.

Accept Your Different Needs and Schedules

It is inevitable that at various points in the process of responding to, and coping with, infertility you and your partner will not be experiencing and feeling the same things, and if you do you may not go through the same things at the same time. So don't expect it. In fact, this is probably a good thing. For example, if your partner's anxiety and stress levels are over the top, it's probably a good thing if you're not feeling as stressed out as she or he is. Likewise, if you're in the depths of depression and despair about your infertility, it's probably better if your partner is not in a similar emotional state. Thirty-five-year-old Kim describes her reaction to her husband's apparent reluctance to pursue in vitro fertilization (IVF) this way:

I wanted so desperately to have my own biological child, and when my husband didn't seem interested in doing IVF, I went crazy. He used to say, "Look, I married you for you, I didn't marry you to have children. We didn't get married to procreate; we married because we loved each other." Now I can really appreciate his words, but at the time I didn't want to hear that he didn't feel the same way I did. I felt terribly alone. Even though he was very understanding, I knew he didn't feel the same way I felt. As it turned out, that was probably a good thing because I would never have been able to stop. I'd lost perspective. I was absolutely driven. In fact, I'd probably still be doing IVF now, still searching for answers, long after it stopped making any sense.

You are entitled to your feelings and so is your partner. Together you will probably provide some balance for each other, and your differences may help you to make more informed decisions that serve you both better in the long run. So aim for mutual understanding and empathy, rather than insisting on emotional conformity.

Also, try to remember that, as women and men, you come to this issue from different vantage points. If you are a man, your connection to having a child is through your partner. She is your link to the procreative process. Without her, having children wouldn't be an issue or a possibility. This means that your relationship with your partner, rather than the product of that relationship, will likely be your first priority. If you are a woman, however, your connection to having a child is through your own body. Your partner may provide half of the genetic material, but the procreative process occurs within you. You possess the potential for creating and carrying a new life within your body. This means that, once motherhood became a priority in your life, it became more difficult for you to disconnect from your own body and your desire to feel a life growing inside you. Thirty-four-year-old Beth describes her frustrations this way:

> *My husband just didn't feel the same way . . . For him it was simple. He said, "I married you because I love you and having children would be a big plus, and if we're gonna have them, that's great, but if we're not gonna have them, we'll just focus on other things in our life." I wasn't ready to hear that because I thought, "Yeah, I married you because I love you too, but I also married you to have children." I wanted both a child and a husband, not just a husband, and I couldn't give up pregnancy and childbirth that easily.*

You both may want to be parents together, but your connection to this process is inevitably different. Try to acknowledge and appreciate this difference.

Learn from Experience

Living with the stress and disappointment and repeated failures of infertility can provide some valuable opportunities to learn how to communicate more effectively with your partner—to learn how to be a better partner. If your relationship is to survive infertility, and even grow stronger through the many challenges, it is imperative that you learn from your mistakes. You need to learn from the inaccurate assumptions, the blaming, the veiled anger and frustration, the avoidance, the threats, the accusations. By stopping to examine the real source of these thoughts and feelings, and by trying to maintain your focus on infertility, not your partner as the problem, you'll have a much better chance of getting through this experience together.

When you find yourself emotionally at war with the person whose child you want to create, you need to listen more carefully to what he or she is saying—without being defensive. You need to try to understand your partner's feelings—without judging. As thirty-eight-year-old Fred found out during his and his wife Eileen's six-year struggle with infertility, relationships can be made stronger if the partners listen to each other and accept each other:

I learned that I had to be more attentive and caring—that I had to just listen to her emotions and let her express what she's feeling . . . I had to be a better listener and just be more patient and loving. I had to learn to be a better person generally . . . that's what I had to learn. That's what going through infertility together taught me.

Keeping Doctors and Everyone Else Out of Your Bedroom

Before you started trying to have kids you probably had a fair bit of pleasure and spontaneity in your sex life. After all, sex was for recreation. It provided a way to be more intimate with your partner. You likely delighted in exploring each other's bodies with the sole objective of giving each other pleasure. Once sex with your partner began to be more focused on the goal of producing a child, however, the purpose of your sexual intimacy shifted from recreation to procreation. Suddenly sexual intimacy had a purpose over and above just pleasure and connection. Unfortunately, this very issue ultimately causes most infertile couples a fair bit of grief and distress in their sex lives.

Initially, goal-directed sex is probably fine—maybe even fun. You're trying to create a child together, trying to take your lives and your relationship to another level. You might even find that sex has more intensity—you're a couple with a mission. However, at some point in the process your intimacy starts to become controlled by the calendar. You start having sex because you're ovulating, not because you're in the mood. Sex loses it spontaneity and becomes regulated. You start listening to other people's advice and old wives' tales about sexual potency. You find yourselves monitoring your alcohol and caffeine intake, having sex in certain positions, and raising your hips (if you're a woman) after intercourse to be sure you're giving the eggs and sperm their best chance to make a connection. Like thirty-one-year-old Jean and her husband, Chris, you might even avoid sex on particular nights in order to save up the sperm so that it's more potent during the times you're ovulating.

If you have sex when you're supposed to have sex, because it's the right time, there's no fun because you're there for a purpose and you're just trying to get a job done. And if, heaven forbid, there happens to be some fun maybe along the line when you're not ovulating, somewhere in the back of your mind you're thinking, "But we're not supposed to be doing it right now. We need to save the sperm—we've got two more days before ovulation!"

After months of not being able to achieve a pregnancy despite your best and most fervent efforts, your sex life, which used to allow you to connect intimately with your partner, starts to become associated with failure. Something that once was a source of pleasure and fun becomes a task that needs to be done at a particular time of the month. You begin to realize that even if you do it when you're supposed to, it probably won't work. You probably won't get pregnant. So you start to ask yourselves, "What's the point?" Sex becomes something you both begin to avoid. After all, who wants to feel like a failure? Thirty-eight-year-old Eric describes it this way:

It starts taking a toll on your sex life. Regimenting sex takes the spontaneity right out of it. I mean, even at the times when you really feel like making love you think, "Oh, the hell with it." After having to perform on command you just get to the point where you'd sooner avoid the whole thing and watch TV.

If this reality isn't enough to completely douse any flames of passion and desire, then the medical investigations and treatment process most likely will be. First, there is the basal body temperature charting, which provides a daily reminder of your fertility problems and the small window of opportunity during the month when you're supposed to have sex. Nicole, a thirty-three-year-old dancer, puts it this way:

I don't think doctors understand how hateful that damn thermometer is. You stick that thing in your mouth every morning and the first thing you say to yourself every day is, "Shit—I'm infertile." It's a hit in the face every morning. And then as if that's not bad enough, you have to circle the number of times you've had intercourse and bring it in so they can check to make sure you're doing it enough. I mean, we had one doctor who told us that our chances of conceiving would be much better if we had sex every night during the middle of the month. At times the pressure was just too much. Sometimes we ended up in an argument and one or the other of us said, "To hell with it . . . just mark the damn circle."

Then, as treatment progresses there are repeated tests and examinations, the majority of which are focused on your genitals and reproductive organs. These procedures can leave you feeling violated, judged, and disconnected from your body and your sexuality. It's pretty difficult to feel good about your body, much less to go home and have spontaneous, uninhibited sex with your partner, after having to masturbate into a sterile cup or having a speculum and catheter inserted in your vagina and cervix.

Making a baby becomes a clinical process, one that isn't even slightly intimate. Eventually it doesn't even require you and your partner to have sex. You don't have to be in the same room together. You don't even have to be in the same building. Ovulation is stimulated by medications, and if conception occurs at all, it happens in a laboratory. Rather than being the product of an act of tremendous intimacy between the two of you, your child seemingly would be the product of science.

Given this shift from sex for recreation to sex for procreation, the association between sex and failure, and the invasiveness of the treatment process, it is not surprising that over time most infertile couples' sex lives become plagued with problems and dissatisfactions. The most common problems reported by couples are related to the loss of sexual pleasure, spontaneity, and desire. Men frequently report difficulties performing on demand, and many experience periods of impotence or instances of premature ejaculation. Sexual problems reported by infertile women include a loss of interest in and desire for sex, problems achieving orgasm, disturbing thoughts and memories during lovemaking (e.g., feeling like they are back on the examination table), and painful intercourse.

When the goal of lovemaking changes from recreation to procreation, and sex becomes work rather than a way to maintain intimacy between you and your partner, some sexual problems and dissatisfaction are inevitable. These problems can be even more severe if you already had some difficulties in this part of your relationship before you began trying to have children. Unfortunately for many couples, sexual difficulties continue to worsen during treatment and seem to persist even after the medical investigations are over, and even if their treatment efforts are successful. Candice talks below about the toll six years of infertility treatments took on her sex life with her husband, Ken.

You know, even now with all that behind us, it's one of the things I feel really sad about. I mean, we've dealt with our infertility and we've become closer as a couple and stronger as people because of it. But we lost something really special because of it. I have such fond memories of the times we used to just play together in bed—we'd laugh and be silly. And there was some great sex as well. But dealing with infertility killed a lot of that. We've never been able to get that passion and spontaneity and fun back in our intimate lives. And that's a real loss for both of us.

Below are some concrete things you can do to nurture this important part of your relationship and keep intimacy alive despite the stresses of infertility. If, despite your best efforts, you find you're still having problems with impotence, premature ejaculation, painful intercourse, or highly disturbing intrusive thoughts during sex, you may want to seek some professional help. A few sessions of counseling can help prevent these from becoming chronic problems and keep them from destroying the sexual intimacy and closeness in your relationship.

Clearing the Room

When you're trying to have a child there seems to be no shortage of misguided, albeit well-intentioned, advice from other people—including respected authors—on what you need to be doing, or could be doing different or better in your sex life, to ensure that you get pregnant. People may tell you:

- "You should have a glass or two of wine before sex so that you're more relaxed."

- "You should have sex every day."

- "You should only have sex in the morning, after you're more rested."

- "You should keep your hips in the air after having intercourse so that the sperm travel up the vagina and don't escape."

- "You should never have sex with the woman on top, because the sperm won't know in which direction to travel."

- "You should save up the sperm for two or three days so that it's more potent."

- "You should wear something very sexy so your partner gets really 'hot.'"

- "You should align the head of the bed with the poles of the earth."

- "You should blacken the windows in your bedroom: chickens, which are prolific breeders, breed in the dark—it might works for humans."

- "You should adopt a child; you'll get pregnant right away."

The advice is endless and, however foolish it may seem at the time, if you're like most couples you eventually try out a few of these suggestions. After all, what can it hurt, right?

Between the well-meaning people giving you advice, and all the medical staff involved in helping you get pregnant, your bedroom can start to feel a bit like a circus. It can get very crowded in there, adding to the performance pressure and stress associated with your sex life. You don't need an audience—even if they're just in your head.

You need to get all of these people out of your bedroom. Once you have charted your basal body temperature for two or three months and your doctor has determined whether or not you're ovulating, remove the thermometer from the side of the bed and take the chart off of your bedroom wall or headboard. You don't need to be reminded of your fertility difficulties every time you try to enjoy an intimate moment with your partner.

Leave the conception issue to the physicians and lab folks since they're the ones with the science and technology, however limited it may be. You may not have control over whether you become pregnant, but you do have control over whether you allow conception—rather than intimacy and pleasure—to become the focus of your sex life. Unless the advice you're acting on would help you enjoy or enhance your sexual pleasure together, then it's probably best to just forget it and try to enjoy yourselves.

Working at Sex versus Sex as Work

It's important to differentiate between the normal changes in sexual frequency, intensity, and satisfaction that occur in most relationships over time, and those that are the consequence of infertility. All couples experience changes in their sex lives; and you probably noticed some changes before beginning your efforts to have a child. Maybe after a few years together you didn't have sex as often as you had previously. Maybe you fell into a particular routine in terms of when and where you had sex, who initiated, and what usually happened. Perhaps you didn't have orgasms as often. Or maybe, as your intimacy deepened and life got busier, you found it didn't matter to you as much whether you had an orgasm every time you made love. Sometimes the connection was enough, and sometimes pleasuring your partner took priority.

These are normal changes that happen in most relationships. As noted above, however, the changes that result from infertility and medical treatment have to do with changes to the goal of your sexual encounters. They have to do with the shift from making love to making babies, and with the sense of failure that you begin to feel each month when a pregnancy doesn't happen. They have to do with "work sex," or sex to achieve a goal.

Unfortunately, a certain amount of work sex can't be avoided when you're trying to get pregnant. There are bound to be times when you have to have intercourse on a particular day, because you're taking fertility drugs, or because you're ovulating—not because you really feel like making love. And if there is a possibility of conception during any of these small windows of opportunity, then it will likely feel a bit like work for both of you. But it doesn't have to feel like work the rest of the time. However, you may have to put some effort into the part of your sex life that isn't about making babies—the part that's about intimacy and love. Frankly, after a while you'd probably have had to do some work in this area anyway, like most couples in long-term relationships, whether or not they are faced with infertility. The following suggestions may help keep your sexual and intimate life more vital.

- Make sexual intimacy a priority.

- Keeping sexual passion and intimacy alive in any relationship requires energy. Basically, you get out of it what you put into it. When you first got together you probably put a fair bit of energy into your sexual relationship. Over time, however, things like work, laundry, groceries, and all sorts of other daily tasks most likely started taking up the energy and space that you once devoted to your sex life. So it's important to make your sexual intimacy a priority again. Put some time and energy into seduction. If you don't, when it happens at all, sex may end up being pretty perfunctory.

- Dare to do something different in your sex life. Give yourselves permission to step out of your comfort zones. For example, you might add body massage or watching erotic movies to your sexual repertoire.

- Incorporate variety in your sex life. For instance, it can help to make love in different places and at different times than usual. For example, if you've fallen into the pattern of having intercourse at the end of the evening in your bedroom, you might consider having sex on a Saturday afternoon in the living room—just to spice things up a bit. You could also change who does the initiating and take turns pleasuring each other, rather than having mutual orgasm as the goal of each of your sexual encounters.

- Get help from a sexual therapist if you need it. If you didn't experience a lot of sexual desire or pleasure before you started having fertility problems, you probably won't have much pleasure now. This may be okay for both of you; not every couple meets their needs for intimacy and connection through sexual contact. However, if you both felt your sex life could have used some attention prior to dealing with infertility, then it would be a good idea to get some help with this *before* you get too far into the treatment process. If you don't, when your fertility treatments are finally over it may be difficult to recapture and build on the intimacy you once had.

Getting Out of Your Head

Two experiences are very common for women who go through infertility. One is that they almost always know exactly where they are in their menstrual cycles, on any day of the month, without having to think about it or consult a calendar. Naturally, this makes it difficult for many women to have spontaneous sex.

So, one of the things you need to do is to stop letting the calendar rule your sex life. Make a point of planning erotic encounters with your partner at times of the month other than when you're ovulating. At first this might be difficult and it might seem pointless. But over time, if you persist, you may come to really appreciate those times when you're connecting with each other in an intimate way, just for the sake of connection, rather than for the sake of trying to make a baby.

The other experience many infertile women have is that, because of the invasiveness of many infertility treatments, while they're having sex with their partners they have flashbacks of being in the examining room with their legs in the stirrups. They have intrusive images of having instruments placed in their vaginas. These invasive images can be very disturbing and certainly can impede any sexual intimacy and pleasure.

While some women may need professional help to deal with these intrusions, many find it helpful to just stop the sexual encounter, and to share with their partners what they're feeling. If this happens to you, you might ask your partner to just hold you and comfort you for a while. You might also use the relaxation exercises discussed in chapter 4 to help you get more grounded in your own body and in the present moment. And by sharing this experience with your partner, he won't be left feeling inadequate or insensitive to your needs.

Staying Connected with Your Body

When you feel like your body has been under assault through all the testing and treatment, and that it has failed you in your efforts to produce a child, it can be very difficult to share this part of yourself with your partner. And yet, there is nothing quite like feeling the gentle touch and caress of someone who loves you dearly, to help heal your damaged sense of yourself and your body. There is nothing quite like being in the arms of someone who loves you unconditionally, to help you heal.

When you don't feel good about your body, try to let your partner help. Tell him or her what you need and what will give you some comfort. If you decide to try sexual intimacy, build on the sexual and erotic activities that used to give you pleasure, and comfort, and joy—the ones that made you feel good about yourself, your partner, and your relationship. As forty-five-year-old Richard says below, the rewards of sticking it out together are worth the effort.

I could never have imagined that an area that had kept us so distant from each other—infertility—and in such pain, could make us feel so close. Infertility has tested us. It has taken us to the edge of despair and has brought us to new understanding and depths, new tightness together as a couple. I wouldn't wish this experience on anyone, but in some ways, it's made us so much stronger . . . When you come out the other end, whether you have been blessed with a child or not, you're different because of having gone through this . . . you're not the same, and neither is your partner or your marriage. If your marriage can survive infertility, it can survive anything!

6

Dealing with Significant and Insignificant Others

Dealing with the stress and disappointment of being unable to produce a child is difficult enough for most couples to cope with. Compounding this difficulty is the fact that it is not easy being infertile in a fertile world. It seems everywhere you turn there are pregnant women or couples pushing baby carriages. Your friends are having children, and some are even having their second or third child. You're feeling out of step. Family gatherings are getting larger as your siblings take partners and have children, and your parents are delighting in their new grandchildren. Colleagues are continually announcing their pregnancies. The world seems geared toward families and as a childless couple you feel that you stick out like a sore thumb.

Being infertile is a silent and isolating experience. It is an experience very few people understand unless they've been through it themselves. Friends and family members are often at a loss as to what to say or how to help. In their efforts to offer support or comfort, they frequently offer advice or say things that make you feel even worse. "Just relax, you're trying too hard." "You need to try harder." "Why don't you quit work?" "Why don't you just adopt?" "You have a good life, why aren't you satisfied?"

Infertility is an experience that also appears to have no clear and appropriate social boundaries. Even people who know you well would consider it inappropriate to ask you how much your mortgage is, how much money you make, or how often you have sex. And yet, when it comes to the subject of having kids, everyone, including total strangers, seems to cross these boundaries without a second thought. As thirty-eight-year-old Dave says below, it's difficult not to get irritated at people who intrude in your personal life in inappropriate ways.

> *We get really annoyed with people who, not out of meanness,*
> *that's not the right word, but out of stupidity and*
> *insensitivity and thoughtlessness, say really hurtful things.*

"Do you have children?" "Why not?" "When are you planning to have children?" "How many children do you plan to have?" Their questions cut like glass. How should you respond? What should you say? What right do people even have to be asking these questions?

In response, you may well find yourself retreating from the fertile world—hurt, angry, and increasingly isolated. But you can't escape entirely. You still have to deal with family, friends, colleagues, and even strangers. You can't do all your shopping after ten o'clock at night when there are no kids in the stores, and you can't avoid every important family or social gathering because it hurts too much to be around babies and young children.

Certainly, periods of isolation have their benefits. They can provide some relief from the onslaught of invasive questions and from the constant reminder of what everyone else seems to have but you—children. Social isolation can close you off, however, from some valuable opportunities to share important moments with people you care about. Isolation can keep you from getting the support you need, so that you don't have to carry this burden alone.

A big part of surviving infertility is learning how to deal with the significant and insignificant people in your lives. Learning how to respond effectively to their advice, comments, and criticisms in ways that keep you from feeling powerless and ashamed. You can set boundaries around the kinds of social interactions you can cope with, and find ways to keep these boundaries from causing misunderstandings and eroding valuable relationships. You can also identify what you need from the significant people in your life, and learn how to communicate this to them. Finally, if you're going to survive this experience with your marriage, your sanity, and your significant relationships intact, you'll need to be able to identify your sources of support, and learn to ask for support when you need it most. The suggestions provided throughout this chapter are meant to help you do just that.

Who Has a Right to Know?

Your desire or ability to have children is not a public matter. It is private—something between you and your partner. It really isn't anyone else's business. However, some people tend to make it their business, when they ask nosy questions or make assumptions that you are selfish or not interested in having children because you aren't yet a parent. Others, like family members and close friends, have more of a legitimate interest in your fertility status, because they care about you. Whether or not you have children tends to affect their lives as well. So you have to decide if you're willing to share this part of your lives with other people, and whom you will share it with.

These decisions will likely depend on three things: the closeness of your relationship, your trust in that person, and where you are in the treatment process. The closer the bond, the greater the likelihood that you'll want to let that person into your private world. This means that strangers, casual acquaintances, and some colleagues may well be left out of the loop, and most probably should be. Unless they are important people in your lives, or unless you have to confide in them because of the demands of treatment (e.g., you have to tell your boss why you need to take time off work), your fertility problems are none of their business. Your task, then, is to decide how to respond to the questions and queries of significant and insignificant others regarding your parental status, without disclosing more than you're comfortable with. Some of the suggestions discussed later in this chapter will help you formulate responses to common questions and comments about your parental intentions and parental status.

Trust is also a really important factor in choosing whom to tell about your infertility. This information is too personal and painful to share with people you don't feel will respond with sensitivity and discretion. Unfortunately, often as a consequence of getting an insensitive response from someone they thought would understand, or finding out that someone violated their privacy by telling someone else, many couples decide to put up barriers between themselves and other people, keeping their struggles and their pain to themselves. The reaction of thirty-one-year-old Anita's mother to news about Anita's recent miscarriage shows how hurtful it can be not to have these losses acknowledged by important people in your lives.

I just couldn't believe my mother's reaction when I told her
I'd had a miscarriage. She knew I had always wanted
children—that being a mother was really important to me.
And yet, when I told her about my miscarriage, she just blew

it off. She said that it happens to lots of women and that I could always try again. Then she said she needed to get some clothes out of the dryer and went downstairs. I was devastated—above all people I thought my own mother would understand.

Although it is unlikely that anyone who hasn't experienced infertility, miscarriage, or the loss of a child will truly appreciate what you're going through, you may have a small circle of people whom you feel you can trust with this information—people who hopefully can provide some support and understanding. Certain friends and family members may fit into this category, while others probably won't. You'll need to make some judgments based on your experiences with these people. Have they shown discretion and sensitivity about private information in the past? Do they refrain from making flippant remarks and comments about other people's problems? Can they be counted on to listen and provide support without giving you advice or dismissing your feelings? Will they accept the choices you may need to make regarding fertility treatments and other parenting options, without judging? If they can be sensitive, respectful, discreet, and caring, perhaps it's worth the risk of letting them in. If they can't, it probably isn't.

Be prepared for the fact that some friends and family members will feel left out, and some may even feel hurt when they learn that you've informed others about your fertility problems but you haven't told them. However, you need to protect yourselves as you attempt to deal with infertility, so your feelings are of primary importance; consider their feelings secondary to yours and your partner's. You'll be in a much better position to respond to their feelings when you've emerged from this and are less emotionally vulnerable and raw.

Finally, your decisions about whom you confide in will likely have a lot to do with where you're at in the process of dealing with your infertility. For example, it is not uncommon in the early and middle stages for couples to keep their difficulties very much to themselves. After all, fertility is so tied up with sexuality and is so connected to feelings of masculinity and femininity that it's not easy to talk about at the best of times. Twenty-nine-year-old Nicholas reflects on this difficulty in the quote below:

I just couldn't bear the thought of telling my family about the fact that we wanted children but couldn't have any because I wasn't able to produce any sperm. I know my dad and brothers too well—everything is a joke to them. I was sure they'd start with the comments about "shooting blanks" and "just let me take your wife upstairs for a few minutes and I'll get the job done for you!" It would have been too much, so I just kept my mouth shut.

The treatment process is invasive enough without others commenting on the details of your intimate life and reproductive functioning. And your infertility may only be temporary, right? So, why talk about something that may not even be an issue soon? Using this reasoning, you may choose to keep your infertility private. However, if you're the type of person who gets a great deal of comfort and support from talking about your thoughts and feelings, and you have people in your life you can trust to understand and be there for you, you may start telling people about your struggles early on. Either way, as time goes on, you may well decide to share your situations with a few significant people. It's usually easier to do so after you and your partner have started to accept the reality of your infertility yourselves and are in the process of exploring other treatment, parenting, or lifestyle options.

Also, as I emphasized in chapter 5, *it is important to remember that this is a couple's issue. Whom it gets shared with needs to be a couple's decision.* It can cause tremendous additional stress in your relationship if your partner feels you have shared this private information with someone else without his or her knowledge or consent, especially if your partner is the one identified with the fertility problem. So decide together who should be told, how much you want to disclose, and when. If by some chance the information accidentally slips out when you're having a conversation with someone—which can happen when you're not at your emotional best—be sure to let your partner know. This will help to keep the communication between the two of you open and honest, and it will help prevent feelings of betrayal from seeping into your relationship.

What Do People Have a Right to Know?

Once you decide you're going to share your struggles with significant people in your life, and you identify the people you are going to share these with, you then have to sort out just how much you're willing to share with them. Do you just tell them that you're trying to have a family, or do you tell them that you're having fertility difficulties? Do you tell them which one of you has been identified with the problem, and what the problem is, or do you keep it vague and let them draw their own conclusions? Do you tell them when you're going through a treatment cycle, or do you wait until the cycle is over and you know the outcome before you let them know what you've gone through? Do you call after the blood test, or do you wait until you see a heartbeat on the ultrasound before you tell them you're pregnant? Do you tell them that the child you're expecting was conceived with the eggs or sperm of someone else, or do you keep this information to yourselves? If you decide to use the eggs or sperm of another family member or friend, how do you keep this information contained so that your rights, their rights, and the rights of your child are respected?

These are difficult questions and there are no easy answers. The reality is that it is much easier to announce a pregnancy than it is to tell people that you desperately want children but may be unable to have any. It isn't easy to say that you're being pumped full of hormones, your eggs are being "harvested," and if all goes well in a few months you might be expecting twins or triplets. It isn't easy to tell people that if you want to have a child you'll have to use the eggs, sperm, or uterus of a stranger.

When you do tell people about your infertility, you'll probably find that most don't know how to respond or how to help. People who haven't experienced infertility usually don't understand what you're going through or the kinds of difficult decisions you're facing. Reproductive technology sounds a bit like science fiction to many people. And third-party reproductive options such as using donor eggs or sperm are concepts that most people have a hard time understanding.

As a result, when you do let people in on your struggles be prepared to do some educating and explaining, so that they understand that babies really aren't grown in test tubes, that using sperm and egg donations to help create a life are not unlike using organ donations to save a life. Know that all of this explaining can be exhausting and frustrating, especially when you're already using all your resources just to cope with treatment and your involuntary childlessness.

If you're using donor eggs or sperm or other third-party reproductive options, the decision whether to disclose this information to others and what you tell them is especially complex. People often have strong moral or religious convictions about these sorts of procedures, and those who care about you may have considerable fears regarding how you and your partner will cope with the fact that only one of you is genetically related to the child. They may worry about whether the child will want or need information about, or contact with, the donor at some point in the future; they may be concerned about whether the child will reject the nonbiological parent. They may be uncertain about whether they'll be able to love the child as much as they would if she or he were genetically related to them. On the other hand, sometimes the important people in your life surprise you, as in the case of Greg, thirty-two:

I wondered, how do I tell my dad that I can't or we can't procreate . . . that if we want kids we're going to have to use somebody else's sperm . . . that if we have a child she or he won't be his genetic grandchild. Like, how could he possibly understand? He's got kids, everybody's got kids. But then after I told him, he just blew me away. He said, "Just do it; go for it. It doesn't matter where your child comes from. We're all God's children, you know!"

Before you disclose this very important information to the other people in your life, be sure to sort out where you stand on these issues yourselves. If you need guidance, refer to the books listed in Resources: these provide very useful information about dealing with the complex issues related to building healthy families through ovum donation, donor insemination, surrogacy, gestational care, and embryo donation.

Overall, when you are deciding how much you tell the significant people in your life about what you're going through, the best rule of thumb is this: Unless most of the people in your social and familial world already know about your fertility difficulties, it's probably best to be judicious in deciding whom you tell, what you tell them, and when. As helpful as it can be to have the support of the people you care about, having to respond to numerous phone calls from people asking, "Are you pregnant yet?" and "Did it work?" while you're going through treatments can add considerably to the pressure you're already feeling. It can also be very painful to face the negative judgments of the people you care about, when you're just trying your best to create a family. So carefully choose those people whom you decide to tell, and be prepared to tell them what you need from them.

Taking Back Your Power: Responding to Insignificant Others

No matter what you choose to do—whether you make your fertility struggles public or not—inevitably you will have to respond to what feel like insensitive, inappropriate, and hurtful questions and comments about your fertility status and your childlessness. It can be very difficult to have to deal with these, especially when you're already feeling vulnerable. However, you may find it useful to reframe these situations as opportunities to help you take back some control and to teach other people about the importance of personal boundaries.

If the comments or questions come from people whom you do not have a close relationship with and who have absolutely no right to be asking these kinds of personal questions, you have two equally good choices:

1. you can simply refuse to answer the question and walk away from the interaction, or

2. you can come back with a response that deflects the speaker's attention away from the topic, or one that puts them in their place and forces them to realize that they've crossed into territory that really isn't any of their business.

Choosing to walk away without offering a response because you've made a conscious choice to dismiss the question and the person asking it can be a great way to deal with the situation—simply not justifying it with a response. However, if you don't respond because you feel caught off guard or wounded by the comment or question, then walking away will likely just leave you feeling even worse. In cases like this it's usually better to have a few pointed remarks ready to use when needed. There are some examples below, but you and your partner may want to put your heads together and come up with a few others that you can pull out when faced with this kind of situation. Rehearsing them a few times in advance can help to make the delivery smoother and more powerful when the time comes to use them.

"Do you have children? Are you planning on having any?"

In response to these very commonly asked questions you might consider saying the following:

"We'd both dearly love to have children, but unfortunately we haven't been blessed with any yet."

This response usually helps people to realize that they've asked a question that is very personal, and if they are at all insightful they might even realize that they've crossed into territory that is really none of their business. To deflect the question without being as obvious about your discomfort with the inquiry you might say:

"We're starting with pets first, to see if we're ready for the responsibility."

"You're so lucky you don't have kids"

When people realize that you've been with your partner for some time and don't have children, they may tell you how lucky you are that you don't have to get up with toddlers in the middle of the night, or spend the whole weekend driving kids around, or deal with obnoxious teenagers. Some may even refer to you as a "DINK," implying that you are a self-absorbed, career-oriented, double-income couple who don't have the time for, or interest in, having kids. These comments and implications can be especially difficult to hear when you'd dearly love to have children and are putting a lot of time, money, and energy into your efforts to have a family—efforts most people couldn't even imagine.

So what might you say in response? To simply shut them down you could say:

"You're right. We have a wonderful life and I wouldn't trade it for anything."

If you want the person to realize that they've made an erroneous assumption and crossed a personal line, you might be more direct in your response:

"You seem to be implying that we don't want children, and that couldn't be further from the truth. Not everyone is lucky enough to be able to have kids, you know."

Or you might say:

"It's easy for you to talk about how lucky we are—because you have your family. Do you really think you'd feel lucky if you didn't have your kids?"

"Too bad you can't have your own children"

We live in a society that values genetic continuity. Inheritance is most often determined by genetic ties, and familial relationships are dictated by biology—whether the person in question is a "blood relative." If you decide to consider adoption or third-party reproduction, you'll likely be the target of insensitive comments that reflect this bias. The experience of Nikki and Peter, a Caucasian couple who adopted a child from China, is a good example of this, as Nikki says:

> When we're out socially with our daughter, it's very obvious that she's adopted. And you can't imagine the number of times people make comments to us, like "It's too bad you couldn't have your own children," or "So you don't have any natural children." It's infuriating, really. After all, this is our "own" child and she is as "natural" as any other child.

Sometimes it isn't worth the effort even to respond to this type of social ignorance. However, if you decide the comment warrants a response, you might consider saying something like the following:

"But this is our own child, and we couldn't love him or her any more than if he or she came from our own bodies."

Or you might say:

"It's too bad you didn't have to work as hard as we did to have your children—if you did you might be more appreciative of how fortunate any parent is to have a child."

Building Bridges of Understanding: Responding to Significant Others

The comments, questions, and hurtful actions of the significant people in your life—friends, family members, and close colleagues—are usually much more difficult to dismiss than those of strangers and acquaintances. These are the people you expect to understand your pain and the ones whose lives you are involved and invested in. That's why their remarks or behaviors, even when they are intended to be helpful, can cut deeply and leave you feeling pretty damaged. The words of Beverly, who with her husband, Harry, finally created their family through adoption, show how family members can inadvertently cause pain by their words or actions:

> My husband's brother and his wife in England had a baby. . . and his mother made a big deal that the mother needed a present too, not just the baby, so she sent my sister-in-law a gold necklace. And yet, when we adopted our child she didn't get me a present. I didn't get a gold necklace because I didn't give birth to this child. I mean Grandma is absolutely thrilled with our daughter and loves her the same as her other

grandchildren, maybe even more because she knows how hard
we had to work to bring this child into our lives. But her
response to how she got here was very different than it would
have been if I'd given birth to her . . . and that really hurts.

When loved ones behave insensitively, your inclination may be
to strike back in response, because you're hurt. Or you may with-
draw emotionally or physically to protect yourself from further hurt.
These are natural responses. However, sharp retorts and emotional
withdrawal often serve only to strain these significant relationships
and make it even more difficult for you to get the support and understanding you need.

Try to remember that these hurtful comments or actions are
most often made out of ignorance rather than maliciousness.
Respond, then, with the goal of facilitating understanding. You can
help the people who are important in your lives to understand your
reality. Yours is a reality that they can't possibly appreciate without a
little help, unless they've lived it themselves.

So, how can you help people understand what it's like to want
so badly, and to be trying so hard to have, something that most people take for granted? Certainly talking directly with the people you
care about, telling them about your feelings and what you're facing,
can be an effective way to build some understanding. But because
infertility is a highly emotional issue, it's sometimes hard to talk
directly without getting really upset. So you might give loved ones
pamphlets or books to read that help to explain what you're going
through (see Resources).

Letter writing can also be a great way to express what you're
going through or let someone know how their words or actions have
been hurtful to you. If you can express your appreciation for what
the person has done, as well as informing them of why you're hurt or
upset, your message will have a better chance of being received posi-
tively. For example, as a way to deal with her pain, Beverly eventually wrote a letter to her mother-in-law. She told her how grateful she
was for the love and support she gave to their daughter. She also
explained how the gift of the gold necklace to the other daughter-
in-law left her feeling hurt. She said she felt less valued for not having given birth. When she opened her Christmas present from her
mother-in-law later that year she found a beautiful gold bracelet with
the word "mother" inscribed on the inside. She had taken a risk in
sharing her feelings and ended up feeling validated and understood
by her mother-in-law in a way she hadn't before.

Like Sherry and Daniel did, by putting your thoughts and feelings in writing, from a safe emotional distance, you can let the people you care about know what you're going through and what you need from them. This also gives them some time to gather their thoughts and sort through their own feelings before they have to respond, and it lessens the likelihood that they'll unknowingly say something inappropriate or hurtful. Sherry describes it this way:

> We sat down together and wrote a letter to our parents. We told them how much we appreciated the things they had done for us over the years, and how lucky we felt to have been raised by such loving parents. We said that they were our role models and that we wanted to be the kinds of parents that they were—and that's why it hurt so much not to be able to have children. We told them we were doing everything within our power to have a family, that we were facing some very difficult choices, and that we needed their love and their support.

Even when you are careful about how and what you tell the important people in your life about your fertility problems, they usually don't know how to respond or how they can help. They may try to protect you from conversations about babies or avoid telling you about someone in the family who is pregnant, for fear that you'll get upset. Or they may encourage you to give up your treatment efforts and just adopt. Or they may tell you that being a parent really isn't that important and that you should just get over it and get on with your life. Below are some examples of how you might respond.

"Why don't you just adopt?"

This question is one of the things infertile couples often hear from well-meaning friends and family members. As important as biological ties are to most people, and as much as pregnancy and childbirth are considered to be significant experiences for women, it is also commonly assumed that adoption is a relatively easy process. Many people believe that because there are a lot of neglected and abandoned children in the world who need homes, infertile couples should quit wasting their time and money trying to have their own biological children and decide to take care of some of these needy kids. If you've been pursuing solutions to your fertility problems for a long time, or you have been putting a lot of energy and money into high-tech treatment, you may very well be asked this question as well.

Your response to this question will likely depend on what you believe the person making the statement means, as well as the situation within which he or she made the comment. On the one hand, if you haven't been sure how your family or friends would feel about your creating your family through adoption, it may be very freeing to hear that they would accept and even welcome an adopted child into the family. In fact, if you're coming to the end of treatment and are getting ready to consider other parenting options, a question like this from the right person can sometimes help you move forward.

On the other hand, if you're not ready to let go of the idea of having your own biological child, or if the question seems to imply that you're being obsessed with, or selfish about, wanting to have your own child, then it can be very hurtful.

So, how can you respond to this question if you're not ready to give up on having your own biological children? If it's a family member asking the question you can simply say the following:

"We're glad you appreciate how important having a family is to us. We aren't ready to move on to adoption yet, and we're not sure that it will be an option we're willing to pursue. But if we do decide at some point to adopt, it's great to know that we have your support."

If the speaker's implication is that you're being selfish in trying to have your own biological children, you might take this approach:

"I wonder how you'd feel if someone told you that you were being selfish to have your own children when there are so many needy kids in the world?"

Or you might consider saying:

"It's hard to consider taking on the special needs of a child who has been abused or abandoned, without first having a chance to see what kind of parents we'd make to a child without these challenges."

Sometimes when significant people in your life suggest that you adopt, their suggestion is followed with the statement *"then you'll probably get pregnant."* The message here, of course, is that once the pressure to become a parent is off, you'll relax enough to get pregnant—or that whatever was blocking your fertility in the first place will get freed up once your maternal juices start flowing. Everyone seems to have a story about someone they know, or the friend of someone they know, who tried for years to have children and as soon as they adopted they became pregnant. Even though there is absolutely no evidence to support the idea that adoption leads to pregnancy, this assumption is still very prevalent. So, you might consider saying the following in response:

"Don't you think it's pretty unfair to bring an adopted child into a home, just so that a couple can get pregnant with their 'own' child?"

"You couldn't possibly understand what being a mother is like"

It's difficult enough to be infertile in a fertile world, but when the important people in your life exclude you from conversations about pregnancy, childbirth, or raising young children, or when they dismiss the comments that you add to these conversations, it can be very frustrating and very hurtful. People may make insensitive comments or exclude you from conversations even when you're an adoptive parent, based on the fact that you haven't experienced pregnancy, childbirth, and breastfeeding. Thirty-seven-year-old Sonya, a physiotherapist whose fallopian tubes were irreparably damaged due to a ruptured appendix when she was in her early twenties, explains it this way:

There is still some disappointment, bordering on anger, that I feel toward friends and family who think I need to be shielded from conversations about childbirth or breastfeeding or taking care of children. They act like I couldn't possibly understand what it's like because I don't have children myself.

Most often, when friends or family members exclude you from these types of conversations, they are trying to protect you from further pain. If they are aware of your fertility struggles and have watched your eyes fill with tears when you've heard the news that someone else in the family is pregnant, they may try to shield you from conversations and situations that might cause you further distress. It's really a no-win situation. If your loved ones include you in these conversations, it can heighten your sense of loss since you can't share your own childbirth or child-rearing stories. If they shield you from these conversations, you can end up feeling even more hurt and left out. That's why it's really important to let the people you love know what you need in these situations.

If, however, when you do participate in these conversations, you feel your comments or advice are being dismissed because you don't have children, or because you haven't been through pregnancy and childbirth, you probably need to address this issue directly. For example, you might consider saying:

"I may not have my own kids yet, but your children are a really important part of my life and I care about them very much."

Or you might say:

"I can appreciate that childbirth isn't easy, but neither are fertility treatments. Between the blood tests, hormone injections, egg retrievals, ultrasounds, and embryo transfers, it's like going through two or three years of labor."

"Why don't you just get over it?"

Initially, most of the important people in your life will likely be sympathetic about your fertility struggles and supportive of your efforts to find a solution. However, after many months or even years of seeing you in pain, they will wonder why you keep putting yourselves through all the drugs, tests, and treatments. Not having been in your shoes, they may wonder why you don't just let it go and get on with your lives.

You may even wonder the same thing sometimes, but when you're not ready to give up your hopes and dreams of growing a life inside your body and seeing the characteristics you love about your partner reflected in your child, these words, spoken by someone you love, can feel like a betrayal. After all, who are they to tell you that it's enough, when they already have their own kids or didn't want any kids to begin with? Who are they to assume that they know what it's like to poke your belly with needles, to pump your body full of hormones, and to give your life and body over to medical science in an effort to produce a child? After all, they haven't walked in your shoes—so how could they possibly know?

The reality is that they can't. The reality is that they don't know how to help. The reality is that it hurts them to watch someone they care about being tortured month after month. They want your pain to end, they want you to be happy, and they want the part of you that was more lighthearted, less serious, and less tormented to return. That's why they want you to get over it—because they want it to end, almost as much as you do. So thank them for their caring and concern, and tell them that you also would like this to be over, but that it's not time yet and that, when it is, you'll let them know because you are really going to need their love and support no matter what the outcome is.

"Thanks, but No Thanks": Responding to Well-Meant Advice

When you let people in your life know that you're experiencing fertility problems, many seem compelled to give you some advice on how to fix the problem. Although these people are probably just trying to help, the underlying message of much of this advice is that you're doing something wrong—that it's your fault that you're not getting pregnant. You'll get sick and tired of hearing it, and it can get very irritating, especially when the person giving the advice is aware that the problem is medical not psychological. And yet, like Jerry and his wife, Jill, after a while you may get a bit desperate and find yourselves acting on some of these suggestions:

> If somebody gives you a piece of advice you almost feel
> compelled to try it out. I still have pictures of my wife
> standing on her head with her hips straight up in the air . . .
> on the advice of a urologist!

So what can you do when you receive unsolicited, albeit well-meant advice? Well, you can simply say:

"Thanks very much, but we already tried that and I'm afraid it didn't work."

Or you might consider saying:

"That sounds like a lot of fun, but I'm not sure the doctors would approve."

One couple I worked with had a wonderful way of responding to these kinds of comments. They would look the person in the eye, smile, and say:

"As it is our sex life is already *very* active. I'm just not sure when we'd fit that in."

Mixed Emotions: Dealing with Other People's Pregnancies and Kids

Dealing with the pregnancy and birth announcements of friends and family members, and being around their children as they grow up, is one of the more difficult aspects of being infertile. These situations are also difficult for your family and friends, who want to protect you from further hurt but don't want to leave you out. Should they tell you they're pregnant, or should they wait until later because maybe by then you'll be pregnant too? Should they include you in their baby showers and family gatherings, or would it be too hard for you to be there? Should they ask you to be godparents or legal guardians of their children, or would that just make you think they feel sorry for you? Should they ask you to attend the birth of their child, or would that only make you feel worse?

And what about you? How should you respond? What is best for you? Is it okay to be told that someone close to you is pregnant, or would you rather not know? Do you want to be told that your sister is expecting a baby, even though you've been trying for years and had hoped to present your parents with their first grandchild? Do you want to be invited to baby showers, or is going to these happy events like torturing yourself? Do you have a right to stay away from family gatherings because it hurts so much to be the only ones without kids? Do you have to say yes to every request to be a godparent or legal guardian? Should you be present during the birth of your sister's, or your best friend's, child? There are no easy answers to these questions, so let's examine them one at a time.

When Someone Else Becomes Pregnant

Would you rather be told that someone close to you is pregnant, or would you rather be protected from hearing this news? As hard as it is to hear that someone else is pregnant, it is usually more painful in the long run to have this information kept from you. After all, you're bound to find out eventually, and it can be much harder to deal with the situation and your reactions when you bump into your friend with her swollen belly or baby carriage. As much as it hurts at the time, it's usually easier to be told sooner rather than later. So when you recognize that your family and friends may be trying to protect your feelings by shielding you from experiences and conversations you might find painful, it's probably best to let them know that it's okay to include you in any pregnancy announcements.

As for your reactions to this kind of news, they will probably be mixed. On the one hand you'll likely be happy for your friend or family member, especially if he or she is happy about the pregnancy. On the other hand, like thirty-six-year-old Casey, you'll probably feel some envy, resentment, jealousy, or sadness because it's them and not you:

I've had a lot of babies being born around me, friends and family members, and it's hard to keep feeling happy for them. I mean, of course I feel happy for what they have, but I can't help feeling cheated myself. I feel almost schizophrenic—one side of me is happy for them and the other hates them for having what I don't have.

Allow yourself to experience these feelings, perhaps expressing them in a journal or when talking with your partner. They are natural reactions to loss, and they will pass.

What about Baby Showers?

Should you hold a shower for your sister or your friend, because you know she'd do the same for you? Should you attend her shower? Attending baby showers can truly be torture when you're infertile. They are events filled with all the joy and promise of new life. The mother-to-be usually looks radiant, and the guests share stories of their pregnancies and birthing experiences. Everyone offers advice on diapers, formulas, and how to get the babe to sleep through the night. It's everything you desperately want, and something that you might never have. And it's even worse when you're in the middle of a treatment cycle, or when you've just had another treatment failure. So the answer to the question regarding baby showers is no—you do not have to attend these events. But you do have an obligation to let your friend or family member know why you can't be there. If possible, talk to her directly. If that's too difficult, then write her a note telling her why you just can't be there and wishing her and her new baby the very best.

Should You Attend a Birth?

Whether or not you decide to attend the birth of your sister's or close friend's child is similar. It is a real privilege to witness the birth of a child. A birth is an incredibly intimate event, one that can draw you even closer together. But, as twenty-nine-year-old Susan says below regarding her nephew's birth, the intimacy and closeness can also be very intense.

Watching him be born was the most awesome experience of my life. It was just incredible. But then I started to get afraid that I would become too attached to him and start putting my nose in where it didn't belong . . . I was afraid of being told that I'm not his mother and that I have no right to interfere. So I've pulled away a bit emotionally and my sister and her

*husband don't understand why. How can you tell someone
that you don't want to love their baby with all your heart
because it's just gonna hurt too much?*

So, you need to decide what you can handle. If you don't feel
you can be there, say so, and explain that you're very grateful for the
offer. If you decide you can handle it, be prepared for the intensity of
the experience, and afterward talk about your feelings with someone
you trust, other than the baby's mother.

What about Family Gatherings and Other Situations Involving Babies?

These same principles hold for other situations that involve
babies, including family gatherings. It's critical that you learn to protect yourself and set some boundaries between what you can cope
with and what you can't. If you let your friend or family member
know why you can't visit her newborn right now, for example, your
relationship will probably survive. Perhaps it might even deepen.
Wendy, a thirty-nine-year-old lawyer who tried unsuccessfully for
eight years to become pregnant, talks about this experience below:

*I'm beginning to be more aware of minimizing the number of
incidents where I could possibly be hurt. I mean every day
there are tons of situations you can come across that include
kids and babies and I'm learning to minimize and protect
myself from some of these. Like my closest friend just had a
baby and I'm dying to get over to see her and her new son,
but I just can't go into maternity wards—this happy place
where there are all these little babies and glowing mothers—it
still hurts me too much, like someone sticking a knife through
my heart. So I can't and won't go see her in the hospital, in
this happy place that I will never be in myself. I'll wait until
she gets home before I go see her. She knows what I've been
going through and she'll understand.*

Family birthdays and Christmas and Easter celebrations are
events that are often geared toward children. When you attend these
as a childless couple you can feel pretty out of place. These types of
family gatherings are often especially difficult events to negotiate
when you're dealing with infertility. There is usually a lot of tradition
associated with these occasions, and if you decide you can't be there,
your behavior may be interpreted as a rejection of the family. And

yet, when you're going through a treatment cycle, or when another treatment has just failed, the idea of attending a family Christmas can be just too much to bear. If you do go and you're miserable, you'll likely make everyone else miserable as well. If you don't go, however, people's feelings may be hurt, especially if those people are your partner's family.

What do you do? You can do one of two things. Either you attend the family gathering, but only for a limited period of time, or you let your partner attend for you and explain to the others why you can't be there. Many couples find that these gatherings get easier to deal with once the children get older and aren't babies anymore, and you might find this to be the case as well. Like thirty-four-year-old Michael, you might even find that you enjoy spending time with the kids and that you can develop a relationship with them without being reminded of what you don't have.

> *I think a lot of the barriers have fallen away now that they're not babies anymore—they're little people and I can talk with them and interact. Their parents aren't so protective and I feel like I can have a role in their lives. It's like finally I have an opportunity to interact with this child a lot more and it starts . . . you're on the path to breaking down those barriers. I go downstairs and play with the kids for a half hour or so and it's great, it's really great. It makes a world of difference. I know it's nowhere near the same as having my own but at least I have that interaction—I get to see the innocence and the sparkle in their eyes and I make them laugh.*

What about Your Role in the Lives of Other People's Children?

Like many infertile couples you may be asked to be godparents or legal guardians of nieces, nephews, and friends' children. In some respects, it's an honor to be asked to fill these important roles. On the other hand, it can feel a bit insulting—especially if you feel the request is being made out of pity. A good rule of thumb to use when responding to these requests is to ask yourselves whether this relationship is close enough that these people would normally be asking you to do this, even if you had kids of your own. If the answer is yes, and you feel that this is a commitment you are able and willing to make, then go ahead and tell the parents that you'd love to be the godparents or guardians. However, if the answer is no, it may be best to tell them that you're honored by their request, but you don't feel that you can say yes, given the other commitments in your life at this time.

Reaching Out for Support

Infertility is not something most couples can handle completely on their own. Maybe for a time you and your partner can weather this storm by yourselves, but eventually you'll need to reach out for support. As thirty-five-year-old Debra says below, after years of dealing with infertility on your own it just becomes more than a couple can handle:

> *We were doing everything alone and it was just too much. We were relying on each other for all our support, and we couldn't keep doing that. We found we couldn't rely on other people in our families to understand. So we started to create a circle of people who were sensitive to what we were going through. They're wonderful and I just know that whatever happens, they are in there with us for the long run. I just know that they will never let us go through anything like this alone—and most of them aren't even family.*

So you need to identify your sources of support. They may be friends. They may be particular family members. Perhaps you'll reach out to other people who are going through infertility as well, or those who have lived to tell about it. Like Simon and Bonnie, his partner, maybe you'll decide to attend an infertility support group (depending on where you are in the process).

> *There was a time when Bonnie wanted me to go to a support group. She was good about giving me some space, but she didn't feel we could keep dealing with this on our own. Eventually she said she was going, and she pleaded with me to go with her. But I just couldn't. I couldn't tell her at the time, but I felt like such a loser—not being able to have kids—and I didn't want to be associated with a whole bunch of other losers. About a year later I did go, though, and it was surprising. All these people were perfectly normal, nice, ordinary people—just like us—people who were just trying to cope with a bad situation, just like us.*

The staff at your fertility center should be able to provide information on local support groups. You can also contact the national office of RESOLVE in the United States or the Infertility Network in Canada for information on support groups in your area (see Resources). These organizations can also provide information on counselors in your area who specialize in working with fertility issues.

Asking for What You Need

The nature of infertility makes it very difficult for people to understand what you're going through and what you need. It is like mourning a death, but there is no body. Each time another treatment fails, another piece of your dreams crumble. It's like a storm that doesn't let up. How do explain that to somebody who hasn't lived it? How do you let people know what you need? And if you do find the words, what if they don't understand? What if you're just exposing yourself to further hurt? In fact, one of the difficult things about being infertile is the profound sense of disappointment and betrayal you feel, when the people you thought would be there for you—the ones you were sure would understand—end up letting you down.

If you are going to get support from other people in your life it is critical that you tell them what you need. For all the reasons discussed above, you can't expect them to know. And how can they know when your needs change, due to new treatments and circumstances? So, in each new situation you're faced with, ask yourselves what you need most—someone to just listen, provide financial support, offer advice, or give comfort—and who might be able to best provide this for you. Then take the risk to reach out to those people, tell them clearly what you need from them, and let them help. Thirty-one-year-old Ann states it this way:

> We haven't really shared our situation with people beyond our very inner circle. We're still in the process of healing. It still hurts every time we have to go and explain it to someone else—I never know what kind of reaction I'm going to get. And I don't need their pity, I need their love. I just need an arm around my shoulder and someone to say, "I don't know how you feel but I'm here if you need someone to listen to you."

7

Hanging On by More Than Your Fingernails: Coping with Infertility over Time

Most difficult and stressful life events are time limited. They happen, you cope with them while they're happening, and then they end. However difficult the situation may be, most people can hang on and weather the storm when there is an end in sight. But infertility is different. When you begin this process you expect it to last only as long as it will take the doctors to identify and fix the problem.

With infertility it usually doesn't work that way. It can take months or even years for your doctors to identify the problem. Sometimes they never find the cause. You begin treatments expecting these medical procedures to work. When the intervention fails you decide to try it again, hoping that the doctors can fine-tune the procedure so that it might work for you the next time. When that one doesn't work, you move on to another. In the meantime you straddle the boundary between the world of those who have kids and those who don't, hoping that in the very near future you'll be able to get on with the next stage of your life—parenthood.

Over time your fertility starts to take up more and more space in your lives. It consumes a tremendous amount of time and energy, emotional as well as physical. It taxes your personal and financial resources. As your investment in finding solutions grows, so too does your commitment. You find it hard to make other important life decisions because your parental status is uncertain—you just don't know if, and when, you're going to be pregnant.

After a while your relationship begins to show the strains of all the stress, the uncertainty, and the months of work sex. This has gone on a lot longer than either of you had expected, and it's wearing you down. You can't remember the last time you really had fun without thinking about infertility, or the last time you and your partner had spontaneous and enjoyable sex—intimacy that wasn't based on the calendar. Sometimes you feel like you're hanging on by just your fingernails. You wonder how much longer you can keep it up without something falling apart—be it your job, your marriage, your health, or your sanity.

What you are feeling is normal. Confronting infertility is like dealing with a life-threatening illness, only in this case the life that's threatened is the life of your potential child (or children). You're doing your best to make the right treatment decisions, you're trying to stay optimistic in the face of some poor odds, and the outcome is uncertain. So how do you cope with the ongoing stresses of infertility during the many months and years that it takes to find answers, pursue solutions, and make alternative parenting decisions? How do you keep from becoming depressed and despondent, and from losing yourself and your marriage in the process? The suggestions in this chapter provide some guidance for keeping yourself and your relationship healthy enough so that, whatever the outcome of treatment, you're in a better position to deal with it.

Moving the Goalposts: Reworking When and How Many Kids

If your vision of the future has always included having kids, you most likely had an idea of when you wanted to start your family, and the age by which your childbearing would be finished. Depending on your family history, and your beliefs about what children need, you may have thought that you'd have your kids while you were younger so that you would have plenty of energy to keep up with them. Or, you may have decided that you'd get your career in order first, so that you wouldn't be as distracted by work or education and could focus more of your time and energy on your kids. Even if you came to the decision to have children later, perhaps in your thirties or forties, you probably felt a need to have your kids by a certain age so that you'd most likely have your health while raising them and be around to see them grow into adulthood.

Everyone has personal goalposts that guide their parenthood decision making—their own internal schedule for parenthood. Unfortunately, infertility usually throws this off, sometimes pretty significantly, which often adds considerably to the stress and distress of this whole process. When you thought you'd be finished having your kids by your early thirties, and you're now pushing thirty-five and still haven't had your first child, it can be pretty frustrating. Not to mention the fact that most of your friends have already started their families, and some have even finished. As a result you probably feel very out of step.

And as if that isn't bad enough, there's also the issue of family size. When you envisioned having kids you always thought you'd have two or three, or maybe even more. But time is passing, neither of you are getting any younger, and you're beginning to feel that you'll be lucky if you have even one child. You're thinking this isn't the way it was supposed to be, it isn't the way your life was supposed to go, and this feeling adds to your sense of urgency for finding solutions. The urgency you feel also affects your treatment decisions. You may decide to go ahead with a treatment cycle you are not emotionally ready for, because you want to have two kids and you're already racing the clock. Or perhaps you decide to skip the less invasive treatment options and move directly to the high-tech interventions, because you feel that you can't afford to lose any more time.

The feeling that this isn't the way it was supposed to be—that you're "off schedule"—also adds to your sense of loss, because even if treatment is successful, it still isn't going to be the way you'd planned it. You're not going to be able to push baby strollers with your best friend when you're both out for your morning run in the park. If you're lucky enough to become pregnant (and probably it's starting to feel more and more like it has to do with luck), your child won't grow up playing with your sibling's children—your child will be several years younger than those kids.

These losses are legitimate, and you have every right to feel disappointed that things haven't turned out the way you'd dreamed and hoped they would. However, it's important not to let these thoughts and feelings have too much weight and push you prematurely, or unnecessarily, into decisions you're not comfortable with. Yes, it's a shame that your children aren't going to experience some of the relationships you'd hoped they would, and that your parenthood schedule is turning out to be different from those of some of your close friends and family members. But in the whole scheme of things, *having* a family is probably the most important issue.

In order to regain a sense of control, you'll need to change your internal goalposts about the timing of parenthood in your lives. These goalposts can become less static and more flexible, so that you have more ability to stay focused on what's really important. Whatever expectations you had about the kind of parent you'd be at a particular age, you need to sort out where these expectations and beliefs came from, work them through, and let them go.

For example, if you're a man in your early thirties who was raised by older parents, you may have always said that you'd do it differently—that you'd be younger when you had your kids so that you'd be energetic and interested in playing ball, fishing, and swimming with them—doing all the things that your parents didn't do with you. However, try to recognize that your sense of what children need comes from your own childhood experience, and that the fact that your parents were older and not as active in your life as you would have liked them to be doesn't mean that you have to be the same kind of parent, irrespective of your age. Think about other men you know who are in their forties or even fifties with young children, and contemplate how much fun they're having with their kids. Settle on an image of one man in your age group who is very actively involved with his kids in the ways you hope to be involved with yours, and make him your role model.

You can also look at the source of your attitudes about the number of children you feel you should have and your ideas of what constitutes a family. For example, perhaps you were an only child and you recall being very lonely or wishing desperately that you had a brother or sister. As an adult, now that your parents are getting older, you still wish you had a sibling to help share some of the caretaking responsibilities and decision making. Because of your own history, then, the idea of having only one child is inconceivable to you. Yet, as your fertility struggles continue you see the years and opportunities for a larger family slipping away, and you find yourself becoming increasingly anxious.

If you are in this situation, you need to recognize the source of your anxiety and of your beliefs about the tragedy of being an only child. Then you need to think about the couples you know who have only one child—try to think of a couple whose child seems well-balanced and happy. What have these parents brought to child rearing that has helped them to do such a good job of raising this child? What have they done to make sure their child has plenty of playmates and doesn't feel lonely? If they could do it, you probably can as well.

"What about My Job?": Fitting Treatment into Your Life

Infertility can take up a huge amount of emotional and psychological space in your life. Between the stress and the hormones, it's sometimes very difficult to think straight, much less maintain any perspective. It also takes up a huge amount of time and energy, especially when you're going through medical investigations and treatments. As hard as you might try to maintain your work commitments, and as much as your work may be a positive source of fulfillment and self-esteem, it can be enormously difficult to schedule all the necessary tests and treatments without disrupting your work life. And it can be equally difficult to schedule your work life around all your tests and treatments.

For example, perhaps you know that you usually ovulate between the twelfth and fifteenth day of the month, but of course you can't predict exactly when ovulation is going to happen. Or perhaps you're going through a cycle of in vitro fertilization (IVF), but your doctors can't tell you for certain when your eggs will be ready to be retrieved. When ovulation begins, or when your eggs reach maturation, you can't postpone your insemination or egg-retrieval procedure for a day or two just because you have a meeting, someone else has called in sick, or you have an out-of-town business trip. If you've been taking clomiphene or superovulation medications, you really can't afford to miss a monthly insemination.

As in the case of Margaret, a thirty-eight-year-old teacher, sometimes letting go of work may seem like the only option.

Every morning I had to drive halfway across the city for blood tests. Then I'd be waiting for a phone call as to how much of this drug to sniff and how much of that one to inject into myself . . . and then there would be the issue of how I was going to mix the stuff and whether there was a private place I could go to do the injections. Then there were the ultrasounds and the inseminations and everything else—not to mention the hours spent waiting in doctor's offices for appointments with physicians and nurses and lab technicians. It got to the point where treatment wasn't just a part of my life, it became my life. I couldn't keep it up—I couldn't protect my privacy and keep taking so much time off work. Everybody kept telling me I had to sort out my priorities—even the doctor and nurses—and having a baby was my biggest priority—so eventually I gave up my job. It gave me more time for treatment, but it also gave me more time to think, and worry, and fret! At least I was good at my job—but I obviously wasn't good at making babies. So I'm not sure letting go of that part of my life was such a good idea—but I just couldn't keep all the balls in the air. Something had to give.

And yet, giving up your job may have some pretty significant consequences. Fertility treatments are very costly. Just paying for the treatments you've already tried, let alone financing the ones that still lie ahead, may be tapping your economic resources even with two of you working.

Also, your work may be one of the few positive things in your life while you're going through infertility. It gives some structure to your days, so that the fertility clock doesn't tick quite so loudly or mercilessly between and during treatment cycles. It gives you a social world outside of the one at the clinic—outside of the world of doctor's faces and nurses and other anxious, stressed-out, and desperate women and men. It may also give you some self-definition and a sense of competence, a feeling that even though you may not be as fertile as some other people, you do have other important skills and abilities. Giving up your work may well mean giving up an important source of your self-esteem and self-definition, leaving far more space for the seeds of failure and incompetence to take root in your self-perceptions.

So what are you to do when you don't feel you can fit everything in? What commitments can you unload in order to relieve some of the stress, without losing a source of positive self-definition? If having children is your top priority, should work be the thing to go? The answer to these questions depends on several factors:

- Is your work a source of positive self-definition, or is it just a job that doesn't mean much to you? If it's just a job, then maybe letting it go will help take some of the pressure off. However, if it's more than just a job, then you might want to think about alternative solutions. For example, you might consider taking a leave of absence for a few months to a year, so that you don't give up your career entirely, but you do make some space for treatment and relieve some of the pressure to perform when you're not up to par. You might consider working part-time rather than full-time for a while. Or, you might negotiate with your employer to reduce the demands of your job for a few months, perhaps taking less demanding cases or projects, or not having as much direct contact with the public.

- Will the financial strain caused by your quitting work actually add more stress to your life and relationship? Will quitting work eliminate the financial possibility of pursuing other treatment options that you feel you need to undertake before you're able to let this go and move on with your life? If the answer is no, then maybe leaving work for a period of time makes sense. However, if the decrease in income will add significantly to your stress, then maybe you'd better consider other ways to reduce the pressure and fit treatment into your life, such as booking the more taxing treatment cycles for a time when the demands of your job aren't as great.

- What are your motivations for quitting? You need to ask yourself if you're buying into the idea that you need to take your fertility, and by association your fertility treatments, more seriously? Are you quitting because you believe that your stress is the reason you're not getting pregnant? If so, then you need to carefully reconsider your decision and challenge these assumptions. What if you give up your work, reduce your stress, and still don't become pregnant? Will giving up a job that you enjoy and that gives you a sense of competence be one more loss in your life when all is said and done? If you give up your meaningful, enjoyable work and you don't become pregnant, what will be left to provide a sense of meaning and purpose and satisfaction in your life?

"What about My Life?": Maintaining Some Balance

As with your work, you'll need to maintain some balance in your life. Infertility and the pursuit of solutions to this problem can become all-consuming. Over time you can get to a point where you eat, sleep, and breathe infertility—where there is virtually nothing left in your life that matters to you or gives you joy and satisfaction. All you seem to be able to focus on is wrestling the infertility beast to the ground. Everything else seems insignificant and meaningless in comparison. You become more disconnected from your partner, from the things that have always given you pleasure, from the other people in your life, from yourself. As thirty-six-year-old Ellen says, after a while you can become obsessed:

I went to the clinic almost every month for three years . . . I was going to succeed at this bar nothing. I was driven . . . if I wasn't doing something, I couldn't stand it. Before I realized it my whole life was around this. I couldn't even take courses or do anything else. Everything was geared toward getting this. I don't know what it was, but I just got kind of driven after a while.

If you are going to get through this experience, it is critical that you not allow infertility to consume you, your marriage, and your life. If you do, and treatment is eventually successful or you become a parent through alternative methods, you won't have much of the joyful, positive person you once were to share with your child. You won't have the stability and strength you'll need in your relationship to face the challenges of parenthood. And if treatment isn't successful, you may be left with only anger and bitterness and sadness, making it more difficult to rebuild your lives together in meaningful and satisfying ways.

So, as thirty-eight-year-old Derek says below, when you spend years trying to have a baby, you'll need to find ways to create balance in your lives—individually and as a couple.

You really have to try to maintain some balance in your life and in your marriage when you go through infertility, because as the time goes on there's a process of erosion, of getting disconnected from things and people that are fun—something you initially didn't have to make a point of doing because you were doing things that were fun. But over time they erode. They get wiped out. Your contacts with people become more disconnected. You become more worn down and it becomes necessary to make a conscious choice to fit things into your lives that are fun—that give you pleasure instead of the constant pain of infertility. If you don't do it, you end up just sort of sinking into a swamp of pain—into a pit of despair.

Although there may be times when treatment cycles are especially demanding and balance won't be possible, you need to be careful not to let your infertility become the primary or entire focus of the rest of your lives. For example, when you feel a sense of urgency to move on to the next round of recommended interventions when a treatment cycle fails, try to stop yourself from jumping right back into the fire; instead, take some time to heal, regroup, and gain a bit of perspective—on yourself, your situation, and your remaining options.

For medical reasons, breaks of at least three months between IVF cycles are usually recommended, to allow your body to return to it's natural rhythms. Emotionally, even more time may be needed between treatment cycles for your emotional well-being, so you can consider the costs, implications, viability, and acceptability of the option recommended next. If you and your partner are not in agreement about the next step, or if one of you isn't quite ready to take that step yet, it's probably best not to proceed with that option. This doesn't mean that you have to stop moving forward; it just means that you need to work through why one partner is uncomfortable with the option in question, and focus on what you need to do together as a couple to reach some resolution on this issue. Perhaps talking it through and giving it a bit of time and space will be sufficient. If not, you may need some professional help to work it through together.

In order to keep the pain and stress of infertility from consuming your life, make a conscious and concerted effort to continue to pursue other interests and activities that make you feel good about yourself and your relationship. You may need to draw on the things that once gave you pleasure, such as art, music, sports, reading, and cooking. If you've stopped buying new clothes because the medications have caused you to put on weight, maybe a new pair of shoes would perk you up. If you previously worked out a few times a week or took dance classes, but you haven't been able to fit these in because of the demands of treatment or because you've been feeling too depressed or lethargic, then you need to put these back into your schedule—at least once a week. Force yourself to go. At first it may be difficult, but once you get started it usually gets easier.

Be sure to incorporate enjoyable activities into your relationship, too. There were likely many things you used to enjoy as a couple—perhaps going to movies, the theater, hiking, boating, skiing, camping. Perhaps these things have fallen by the wayside during the years you've been trying to become pregnant, and maybe some of the people who used to join you in these activities now have children and are no longer as available. Or, perhaps when you do go out together for a meal and a movie, you end up talking about your infertility and childlessness, causing you to just get more depressed or fight with each other.

Make a point of doing some of these activities together at least once a week—activities that you both enjoy. Declare these brief respites "infertility-free zones"—times when you talk with each other about other interests and events in your lives.

Before they started dealing with infertility, Peter and Linda turned down all invitations to social gatherings and events on Friday evenings. They'd come home after work, grab a pizza and a bottle of wine, climb into bed with a good movie, and refuse to answer the phone or let the world intrude on their privacy. They stopped doing this for a few years when they were first dealing with their infertility, but they decided that they both missed these quiet evenings together very much. So they reinstituted their policy of keeping Friday evenings to themselves, and in the process they rediscovered how to connect with each other in a satisfying and meaningful way.

Infertility as Part, Not All, of Your Identity

Just as infertility can take up a lot of space in your life, over time the focus on treatment and the constant failures can begin to take up a larger portion of your identity. When someone tells you that you can't produce a child, while thousands of children are conceived every year by parents who either don't want them or can't care for them, it's hard not to feel like there's something wrong with you. Or when a physician tells you that your eggs or sperm are of "poor quality," or that your tubes are damaged beyond repair, or that your ovaries are "failing" to respond, it's very difficult not to take the failure of your body personally, not to see yourself as a failure.

That's why it's so important that you maintain some balance and perspective and not let your infertility totally define your sense of who you add up to as a person. You may be dealing with infertility but you are more than just the sum of your fertility status, and so is your partner. You are not just an infertile man or woman; you are not just an involuntarily childless couple. You have other roles and interests in your life that also define who you are—daughter or son, lover, partner, friend, worker, artist, or dancer.

So rather than letting infertility and a sense of failure consume and define you, identify your other valued roles, and try to rely on these to sustain your self-esteem. One way to do this is to sit down with a piece of paper. On the top of the page in bold letters write the words "Who am I?" Then, write the numbers one through ten down the left side of the page. Next to each number write the words "I am . . . " and finish each sentence with a word that represents a different role in your life. In my case, I would likely include my work roles of university professor, psychologist, and writer. I might also include my relationship and family roles of partner, friend, mentor, and daughter. And I might include in this list particular traits that I value in myself, such as loyalty and commitment.

Try this exercise. See if you can come up with at least ten words that describe who you are. Perhaps you'll come up with even more than ten. If you can't seem to gain any clarity or perspective on this, then ask your partner or other people who know you well what they see as your strengths and your gifts. Don't let roles or characteristics related to your infertility or parental status take up more than a space or two.

Once you've compiled the list, try to put the items in the order of what you value most about yourself. Then, draw a circle and divide it up proportionally like a pie, based on the amount that each of these roles, traits, or characteristics defines you. Write the appropriate description in each section. Hopefully you'll see that infertility is only one part of who you are, even though it feels so completely defining at times. Then take this circle and put it someplace where you will see it on a regular basis, perhaps on your refrigerator door or on the mirror in your bathroom. When you start feeling that infertility is closing in and consuming you, take a look at this circle and try to remember that you add up to far more than the sum of your infertility.

Dealing with the Ongoing Ambiguity of Your Parental Status

One of the more challenging aspects of infertility to deal with is the continuous uncertainty of your parental status. You don't really fit into the category of people who are parents or who are making the transition to parenthood. On the other hand, you don't fit into the category of those who are voluntarily childless. Your world and decisions are based on constructing a meaningful life with children, not as a childless couple. But your plans are already way off schedule and at times you're not even sure you'll ever become a parent. At the very least, the transition is taking an inordinately long time and in the meantime you still have a life to live.

Essentially you're stuck between these two worlds as you try to become parents; meanwhile the ambiguity of your parental status can persist for months and even years. Kevin, a thirty-seven-year-old chiropractor, refers to it this way:

I think what is most difficult is that we keep going and having tests and treatments and nothing works. I mean if they could just tell us they can fix the problem or they can't fix it, then we could deal with it and could continue from there. But they can't. They just keep saying, everything looks good, it's just a matter of time—of finding the right treatment. And where does that leave us? Absolutely nowhere! Like now what? It makes it pretty hard to get on with our lives. In fact, it makes it impossible! Here we are, four years later and we're no further ahead—no closer to being parents.

It is this uncertainty—this sense of being stuck, of not being able to plan your lives—that makes coping with infertility especially challenging. If you knew that you weren't going to be able to have children, it would be difficult, but you would find a way to deal with that reality and begin to make decisions about the rest of your lives. You'd rework your priorities and set new goals based on a life without children, or you'd get on with finding another way to become parents, perhaps adopting locally or internationally.

However, as long as there is still a possibility that you might become pregnant, it is very difficult to plan your lives. Making basic life decisions, such as knowing where you want to live, what size vehicle you need, and what types of jobs you want, can be pretty challenging when you don't know whether or not your future is going to include children. For example, you may be thinking about buying a new car. But should you get a small two-door vehicle, something sporty and fun, or should you buy a larger, four-door car that can easily accommodate a child car seat in the back? You may be considering a move to a new home or neighborhood. But do you buy a two-bedroom condo in an urban neighborhood close to where you work, or do move to a larger home in a family-friendly neighborhood, close to good schools? You may have an extra room in your home that needs renovating. Do you turn it into a home office now or do you wait until you know for sure whether you're going to need it for the nursery? Maybe your boss has offered you a new position that you've always wanted, but the job requires a fair bit of travel. Do you take the job and fit infertility treatments around your travel schedule, or do you say no to this promotion, knowing full well that the opportunity may not come around again? Perhaps your partner has been asked to relocate to another part of the country, a promotion that will make it much more affordable for you to stay home for the first few years when you have children. But you've been on an adoption waiting list for over two years and if you move you'll lose your place on the list. Do you agree to the move?

When your fertility status is so uncertain and you don't know whether you're ever going to become parents, you can find yourselves feeling pretty paralyzed when faced with these types of decisions. And yet staying in this holding pattern can add considerably to the feelings of powerlessness and depression that are so often a part of the experience of infertility and medical treatment. You can find yourselves several years later, having put your lives on hold and having devoted your financial and emotional resources to trying to have children, not only childless, but also having passed up important opportunities for personal and perhaps professional growth. Lisa, a forty-two-year-old college teacher, describes it this way:

> *I look back now and think, God, we were in such a holding pattern for so many years. I think about all those lost years—years when we were so focused on trying to have a baby that we missed out on so many other things. I don't regret that part, the trying part. It was really important that we tried everything we could to have our own biological children. I have no regrets about that part. But I do regret the lost relationships, and the lost opportunities. It didn't have to be that way, but at the time it's like you're caught in this vortex and everything seems tied to having kids—like you have kids or you pursue your career, you have kids or you travel. And yet it really didn't have to be either/or, it could have been both. But we didn't see that then, and that's what I really regret.*

When you're going through infertility and pursuing treatment, everything seems to hinge on whether or not you have kids. And yet, as Lisa says above, it doesn't have to be that way. The costs in terms of lost opportunities and lost relationships can be even higher if all your decisions are framed in this either/or way. Choosing to have children is an irrevocable decision. Once you have a child there is no turning back—you'll always be a parent. However, most other decisions in life, however significant they may be, are not irrevocable. Knowing this can help you take your life "off hold." If you buy the two-seater sports car and end up getting pregnant, then you can trade it in later for a family vehicle. If you turn the extra room in your home into an office, you can make it a nursery later, if your efforts to have a family are successful.

Of course, you should pursue whatever options you feel are necessary to ensure that you won't have regrets later. However, when making other important decisions in your lives, *you need to base these decisions on factors other than your possible future parenthood.* In fact, as difficult as it may be, *you need to base these decisions on what would be best for you and for your partner in terms of your personal growth and your growth as a couple,* rather than on whether or not you're going to have kids. By making these your criteria for your decision making, you are more likely to have the strength to cope with biological childlessness, if treatment fails. And if treatment succeeds, you'll bring a healthier sense of yourselves as individuals and as a couple to your new role as parents.

For example, let's say you are a woman who has been working for several years at a job that hasn't been especially challenging or satisfying, and you really need a change. You've needed a change for a while, but you've been hanging on because you hoped to be pregnant soon and planned to take a few years off work to raise your kids; perhaps you have a better career in mind, and you've planned to go back to college after your kids start elementary school. You've been in this holding pattern now for a few years and don't feel especially good about your job or about your reproductive abilities. When you think about starting college now, you wonder whether you have the time or emotional energy that the course work would require. After all, with the fertility drugs and all the stress, you figure you probably wouldn't be able to concentrate or think straight. After so many months of treatment failures you don't have a lot of confidence in yourself, and you wonder if you even have what it takes to pull off decent grades. Besides, if treatment is successful and you do become pregnant, you'd have to stop taking courses for a while anyway, so what's the point of starting something new now?

The point is, you need a change and a challenge. You need to invest your energy in something that makes you feel good about yourself and helps you build a vision of the future that is more promising. You may indeed become pregnant in the next few months, but you might not. And the years are going to pass anyway. If you do become pregnant, you can decide at the time whether to stop taking courses, depending on how you feel during your pregnancy and after the baby is born. You can always start your courses again later, if and when you're ready. And if you don't become a parent in the next few years, you'll be that much closer to a meaningful and satisfying career.

Getting out of the holding pattern that infertility and the pursuit of parenthood have imposed on your lives can ultimately make it easier to cope with the stresses and failures of medical treatment. *Getting on with your life does not mean you're giving up on having children. It means you care enough about yourself and your relationship to be sure that both are as healthy as they can be, under the circumstances.* You can't control your fertility, but you can control the choices you make about the other important things in your lives. So if you find yourselves having difficulty making a decision because of your uncertain parental status, ask yourselves the following questions:

- Is this something I/we feel good about?

- Will this be good for me personally and/or for us as a couple?

- If I/we don't do this, and we don't end up becoming parents, will I/we likely regret it?

- If I/we do this, and we end up becoming parents, does it really matter?

If your answers to the first three questions are "yes," then it's probably worth taking the risk. Because most likely, should you happen to become parents after you've made life-affirming choices for yourselves, you'll still be able to fit kids into your life—you'll just be fitting them into a life that is full and rich, rather than one that has stagnated from too much frustration, failure, and loss.

Not Letting It Wear You Down

It is extremely common after months or years of dealing with infertility to feel tired, exhausted, emotionally flat, low energy, apathetic, and downright depressed. This is understandable. The physical and emotional demands of medical testing and treatment alone can place tremendous pressure on you and your partner, especially over a prolonged period of time. Added to this is the fact that going through infertility is like riding an emotional roller coaster, with the highs coming at the fertile point in your menstrual cycle or at the point of treatment intervention, and the lows following two weeks later when you realize that again you're not pregnant. Having to be on this ride for a short period of time would be challenging enough for most people. But being on it for years is bound to wear you down.

Compounding this exhaustion are the repeated losses you feel when you're infertile. The tragedy of being unable to produce a child is like the tragedy of losing a child. You have a dream of the type of parents you're going to be and of the type of child you're likely to create together. And each time treatment fails, it's a bit like losing that child. Each time you have another menstrual period, the child you'd hoped for seems to slip further away. Such a loss, felt over and over again, is bound to make you feel sad and cause you grief. And people who are grieving usually experience low energy and feelings of depression.

If you find yourself in this situation, consider the following things:

- Understand that your reaction is a normal reaction to loss, and try not to expect too much of yourself. After all, if someone you knew had just lost their young child, you wouldn't expect them to be coping well. You wouldn't expect them to just get over it, so don't expect that of yourself. The only difference here is that yours is the loss of a dream, a progressive loss that you've been living for many months or even years. Putting your experience in this context can help you, your partner, and the significant people in your life set more realistic expectations for what you are capable of handling.

- Be aware of the tremendous toll that prolonged stress, repeated losses, and infertility treatment has taken on you. In fact, even when women become pregnant after years of infertility treatments, it's not at all uncommon for them to feel emotionally drained, physically exhausted, and perhaps a bit depressed, even though they're thrilled that they're finally pregnant. This is because they still have to recover from the residual emotional and physical exhaustion from the treatment process and from the uncertainty they've been living with for so long.

- The demands of going through infertility are not unlike the demands of running repeated marathons. At the end of a race runners are physically and emotionally exhausted. They need time to replenish their energy, tend to their bodies, and refocus their minds, before they race again. Treatment cycles are similar. After a failed cycle, you need to take care to replenish your emotional energy and attend to your overall mental and physical health. Eat well, even if you have no appetite. Get some exercise, even if you have no energy. Focus your thoughts on things that make you feel good about yourself, rather than on your sense of failure. And take the time to express your feelings of sadness, loss, and grief—by talking, writing, or perhaps by creating art. One woman I know, though not an artist, painted pictures as an outlet for her emotions during her infertility experience. Now an adoptive mother, she looks back on these pictures as a chronicle of her journey to parenthood, as validation that she's earned the right to revel in every detail of her young daughter's growth and development, and as a testament to her own strength and resourcefulness from having survived such an exceedingly difficult experience.

- If you find that you're having difficulty getting out of bed in the morning, you're crying all the time, you can't concentrate on anything, and you're unable to keep up with even basic tasks at work and/or at home, you need to see your family doctor. It is possible that your symptoms are not just the result of your fertility struggles. Rather, you may be suffering clinical depression, in which case a brief course of antidepressant medication and counseling might be necessary to help you get through this difficult period.

Viewing Your Body as a Friend Not a Foe

Because infertility is a loss associated with the physical inability to produce a child, if you've been told your sperm aren't capable of fertilizing your partner's eggs or that there are problems with your eggs, fallopian tubes, uterus, or hormones, it is difficult not to believe that your body is inadequate. When you can't produce a baby, it's hard not to feel like your body has failed you.

Part of the problem is that medical treatment, with its focus on body parts and tests and procedures, sets you up to feel like you either pass or fail. Either your sperm has "good" volume, motility, and morphology, or it "fails" to meet these standards. Your hormone levels are "normal," or your ovaries are no longer "receptive to stimulation." Your eggs are able to be "fertilized," or their quality is "deteriorating." Your embryos are "excellent," or they are "poor quality." Even if you are in very good health overall and take excellent care of yourself, the implications and language associated with medical assessment and diagnosis can contribute substantially to your feelings of physical inadequacy and failure. Add to this the fact that fertility drugs can cause weight gain and bloating and it becomes even more difficult for you to like, or be comfortable in, your body.

Another factor that contributes to these feelings of bodily betrayal is the reality that fertility is highly valued in our society. It is closely tied to perceptions of masculinity and femininity. Your body's inability to reproduce or carry a viable pregnancy, then, can seem like an assault on your sense of your masculinity or femininity.

This sense of your body having failed you can play itself out in many ways. For example, you might find yourself paying less attention to your appearance or how you dress. You might let your eating habits go and stop paying attention to your level of fitness—unfortunately only exacerbating your dislike of your body. Or, your feelings might be more localized. If you're a man who isn't able to produce sperm, you might find you experience periods of impotence. Or, if you're a woman whose uterus seems unable to carry a viable pregnancy, you might feel that the monthly reminders of this failure are too much for you to cope with and find yourself asking your physician to perform a hysterectomy. You may feel that the inconvenience of having periods isn't worth the trouble if you're probably never going to be able to carry a child anyway.

While these feelings are entirely normal and understandable, they usually end up making you feel even worse about yourself and your situation. Instead, try to focus on the many other critical functions your body performs in your life. Try to focus on what your body can and does do, rather than on what it can't. Force yourself to consider your physical strengths, perhaps your sturdiness, athletic ability, excellent vision, sharp memory, strong hands, lovely hair, or beautiful eyes. When you start to feel disenfranchised from your body because of its inability to achieve a pregnancy, try to focus on these strengths, rather than worrying about whether your sperm are swimming properly or your eggs are able to be fertilized.

You also need to find ways to separate your fertility status from your sense of masculinity or femininity. Just as a woman who loses a breast to cancer or a man who loses his testicles isn't less feminine or masculine because of the loss of a body part, you are no less feminine or masculine because of your infertility. It's fine to hate your situation, but hating your body for what it can't do only adds to the casualties of your infertility.

Living between Two Worlds: Preventing Social Isolation

Another difficult challenge of infertility is that it is a socially isolating experience. Many of your friends may have already made the transition to parenthood and are now less available for social gatherings. Even if you and your friends still share a common interest in certain activities, like playing a sport or going to the theater, they certainly aren't as free to do these things as they were before. And, because raising young children is a primary focus of their lives now, when you do get together you find you don't have as much in common as you once did. Furthermore, unless they've been through infertility themselves, they probably can't relate to what you're going through or the types of choices you're facing. And yet, because infertility and fertility treatments are a large part of your life right now, it's hard not to talk about what you're going through, and it's even harder when people don't really understand. As thirty-four-year-old Terry says below, being infertile can be very isolating:

> At times I know I should just come out with it and say what I'm feeling and what's bothering me but it sounds so much like the same old story, same old, same old, same old. So I don't end up saying anything—I just keep my feelings to myself, more and more. No one can sympathize anymore because they keep expecting the problem to be resolved, but for me isn't resolved—I'm still not a mother.

So how do you deal with the isolation? How much time do you invest in your relationships with friends and family members who have young kids, especially given how hard it is to be around people with babies? And yet, you might be parents yourselves one of these days and these are people with whom you'd likely enjoy sharing your parenthood experiences. How do you keep from being socially isolated while also protecting yourselves from too much frustration and pain?

It is best not to break your ties with the important people in your lives, just because they have children and you don't. Yes, it may be difficult to listen to them talk about the trials and joys of parenthood. And you may not be able to count on them to understand your reality or be as available as they once were. But if you are successful in your efforts to become parents, these relationships may become even more important. And if you don't become parents, once their kids are a bit older, they might have more time to invest in common interests, and you might enjoy and appreciate spending time with their kids.

So, if the relationships are important to you, try to maintain some contact, although it may be more limited than it was before they had children. If being around their young kids is too difficult for you, try to center your social time around activities or events that you can do together as couples, while a sitter watches their kids. Limit your contact with their kids to significant events, like Thanksgiving or their children's birthdays, and don't stay too long if you're finding it painful to be there. Or perhaps one of you can put in an appearance on your behalf so that your friends know you appreciate the significance of the event in their lives, and so that you don't cause yourself further pain.

Try to develop a social network of other childless couples with whom you enjoy spending time. It can be very helpful if some of the couples in your social network haven't yet had children or aren't planning on having any. However, if you don't have many childless friends, then you need to try to cultivate a few of these relationships, perhaps based on a shared interest. You may find that investing a bit of time and energy in these relationships keeps you from feeling quite so socially isolated and out of step with your other friends. Be clear about and accept these relationships for what they are, though. If they are based on a shared interest in a sport or activity, then that's what they contribute to your life. They may not ever evolve into something deeper or longer-lasting. But if they help you stay involved in things that are of interest to you, distract you from your infertility if only for brief periods of time, and keep you from the increasing social isolation that is so common among infertile couples, then they are more than worth the effort and investment.

As discussed in chapter 6, people who have children and those who have never wanted children often can't appreciate what it's like to experience infertility. They don't usually understand the types of difficult decisions you face in trying to create your family or the phenomenal stresses involved in treatment. As a result, you may find that you are not able to talk openly and candidly about your infertility with most of the people in your social world. If this is the case, and you feel a need for some support besides what your partner is able to provide, then you need to seriously consider joining a support group. Those who have also lived this experience know only too well the depth of your pain, the extent of your struggles, and the degree of your investment in trying to have a child. Having been through the experience, they are usually able to provide a shoulder to lean on, without insisting on giving advice. Often they can provide information about the local health-care providers as well as the available treatment and parenting options. Even if your partner isn't interested in attending support group meetings, you may find that you benefit from going by yourself, rather than trying to deal with infertility on your own. Ask your physician for information on local support groups, or contact the head office of RESOLVE in the United States or the Infertility Network in Canada (see Resources). Or, you may find it helpful to access the support of other infertile women and men through infertility Internet newsgroups such as www.alt.infertility and www.misc.health.infertility.

"We Need a Vacation": Taking a Break from Infertility

After a while, infertility can begin to consume you, and the prolonged stress can wear down your physical and emotional resources, and take a toll on your relationship. So it is important to find ways to build breaks from infertility into your lives. I realize that this is easier said than done; as long as being parents is still your central goal, and your parental status remains uncertain, you can never completely leave infertility behind—it is always there. But it doesn't always have to be front and center in your lives and in your minds. You can make a decision to put it on the "back burner" while you put a bit of time and energy into other parts of your lives and relationship.

For example, you may have an insemination booked but find that you're feeling overwhelmed by other demands in your life. Give yourself permission to skip the cycle and do it the next month instead. Or perhaps you have a vacation planned and it turns out you're going to be ovulating during the time you planned to be away. Make the decision to go on your vacation—when you come back you'll likely be in a better state of mind to deal with the stress of another treatment cycle. Or, you may have just finished your third cycle of IVF and are now considering a third-party reproductive option if you're going to achieve a pregnancy. Instead of starting treatment immediately, let your body heal a bit, take some time out to regroup and reconnect with your partner, and consider what you're most comfortable pursuing. In so doing, you'll be more likely to make the kind of decision that you'll be satisfied with in the long run, and you and your relationship will be in better shape to deal with all that another round of treatment involves.

8

A Fight Well Fought: Deciding It's Time to Move On

If you are still pursuing medical solutions to your fertility problems perhaps months or years after you expected this process to be over, you are faced with a very difficult challenge—deciding when it's time to give up the fight to have your own biological child and get on with the next stage in your lives. It's very hard to know when you've done enough, when you've had enough, and when you can walk away without regrets. As Mark, a forty-one-year-old pilot, points out, it's hard to know whether having children just wasn't meant to be:

> We used to talk about feeling like guinea pigs on the wheel in a cage. Once you get on, how do you get off? Every move you make, you just go faster and the wheel doesn't stop—it just doesn't end. Eventually you have to find a way of just jumping off in mid-flight to stop it. You go through this emotional roller coaster and you get all excited and then it bombs, and then you get all excited again and it bombs. We did that for eleven years. I mean, at some point you've just got to say, "It just wasn't meant to be."

It's very hard to acknowledge that biological childlessness is meant to be your permanent fate. It's frightening to face the thought of a future that might never include children. That's why, even when your doctors say they have nothing left to offer you, you may insist on trying in vitro fertilization (IVF) "just one more time"—and that's why one more time ends up being two, three, or four more times.

Compounding this difficulty is the fact that you and your partner may not get to this point in the process at the same time. One of you may be ready to throw in the towel and move on, content in the knowledge that you've given it your best effort and anxious to regain some sense of normalcy and joy in your life and relationship, while the other is still committed to trying one more round of treatment, or as many rounds as it takes to become pregnant.

You and your partner may in fact agree that you're reaching the end of the line, but actually stopping may not be that simple. With hope fading and no other options to consider, you may both resolve that this is definitely going to be your last treatment cycle. You agree that if it fails you'll both feel content with the knowledge that you've done everything possible to try to have a baby and that you can then move on. Your resolve may be challenged, however, when in his or her honest efforts to help after a failed treatment cycle, your doctor suggests that there might be one more treatment option worth trying, igniting the flames of hope again.

As you've come to realize only too well, hope can be a double-edged sword. On the one hand it can prevent you from hitting the wall and having to deal with the full impact of permanent biological childlessness. On the other hand it can keep you involved in an endless pursuit of answers and solutions. It can keep you locked in a holding pattern even when the odds of success are so remote that they couldn't possibly justify the investment of more time, money, and effort. And yet, however illogical it may seem, you may fear that if you don't try the treatment in question, you might regret it later. Renee, a thirty-five-year-old paramedic with unexplained infertility, puts it this way:

> I think sometimes the physicians do a disservice by building
> up hope, and suggesting that maybe one more treatment or
> some fine tuning of the last treatment just might do the trick.
> The disappointment is so much greater when these hopes
> aren't realized. I mean, it's nice that they're trying to help by
> suggesting another treatment, but I kind of wish they
> wouldn't, because it's like, we get to a point where we say,
> "Okay, this is the last thing left to try and then we can
> stop—we can get on with our lives." But then when it doesn't
> work, they suggest something else and we get hooked in again.
> I mean, they hold out another possibility and it's like, if we

don't make use of this opportunity will we be able to live with ourselves? Will we regret it? Will we always wonder if maybe that would have been the treatment that we finally got pregnant on?

When Your Treatment Efforts Are Successful

If your treatment efforts are successful and you end up with the pregnancy you've hoped for and dreamed of, answering the question of when to move on is relatively easy. However, you may well be surprised at the emotions you end up experiencing when you realize that you're finally pregnant, ranging from surprise and delight to fear and anxiety. These are normal feelings, given the tremendous emotional investment you've made in trying to have a child. You're bound to feel plenty of anxiety about this hard-earned pregnancy, about whether everything is okay.

Even people who haven't been through infertility usually experience anxiety during their first pregnancy, wondering if the baby is healthy and if they are up to the challenges of raising a child. No matter how strong the desire to have children, there is always some fear and anticipation associated with the tremendous life changes that parenthood inevitably brings. The knowledge of how hard you have worked to become pregnant in the first place, and how difficult it might be to become pregnant again if anything goes wrong with this pregnancy, adds to your anxiety.

Overall, however, the joys of finally making the transition to parenthood will probably outweigh your fears and anxieties. You'll likely feel very grateful to the medical staff who saw you through this difficult time in your lives and helped make your dreams of becoming parents come true. Your focus will shift to planning for your future as a family, something you weren't able to do for so many years. And you'll be very relieved to close this chapter of your lives, at least temporarily. Whether you're finding yourself elated or anxious about being pregnant, you may find Ellen Glazer's book *The Long-Awaited Stork* (1990) to be a helpful resource for information on how to cope with the unique stresses, joys, and challenges of pregnancy and parenting after infertility.

How Do You Know When It's Time to Move On?

Deciding that it's time to quit when you haven't been able to become pregnant, however, is often very difficult. It is a conclusion that different people come to in different ways depending on a range of factors, including their values and personalities, their available financial and emotional resources, the state of their relationship, and their ability to envision a satisfying future without their own biological children. It is a very personal decision. No one, not even your partner, can tell you when it's time to quit. It's an individual choice, one that no doubt will be influenced by your partner's wishes, but inevitably the resolve to move on must come from deep within each of you.

So how *do* you decide that you've done enough? How do you know when it's time to give up the battle and abandon your treatment efforts? How do you know that you won't have regrets later? And, once you do give up the fight, how do you cope with the grief and loss, make decisions about the other available parenting options, and create a new vision of the future—one that may or may not include children? These questions are addressed in this chapter. Let's begin with the first step: realizing that you've had enough.

When Desire Turns to Desperation

Although there are no clear criteria that work for everyone in coming to the decision to abandon their treatment efforts, there are some common signs that the time has come. One strong indicator is when your desire to produce a child turns to desperation. This is usually most obvious in the way you make decisions about treatment.

When faced with a treatment decision your desire to produce a child is usually balanced with some assessment of the odds, combined with an intuitive sense of what you can live with. However, your desire has probably turned to desperation if you find yourself making the decision to do one more treatment cycle, however remote the probabilities of success, without any thought about the costs or consequences of doing so—to yourself, your body, your relationship, or even the child that may be produced. The following quote by Allissa, a thirty-seven year old actress who, after three years of trying to become pregnant, was diagnosed with severe endometriosis, is a very powerful example of how desire can turn to desperation:

Following several years of medical investigations, my physician informed me that extensive surgery would provide my only hope of conceiving a child. My immediate response was, "Book it." "But don't you want to know what it involves?" said the physician, to which I responded, "Book it." "But don't you even want to know the probability of success or the risks?" said he. I implored him, "Please, just book it." At that moment, I realized that had the physician told me women with one leg have a better chance of conceiving a child, I would have unhesitatingly offered to have my leg cut off. I knew then that it was time to quit . . . that it wasn't making sense anymore.

You'll know that desire has turned to desperation when:

- the possibility that you've come to the end of the line is so intolerable that you can't even allow yourself to consider it

- you are told that the treatment has a 95 percent chance of failure, and you focus only on that 5 percent chance of success

- you find yourself pleading with your physician to let you try one more round of treatment when she or he has indicated that there is nothing else to offer you that has even a remote chance of succeeding

- you start looking for other clinics to offer you a treatment that your doctors feel is futile or harmful

- you find yourself considering treatment options that you know your partner is opposed to, and ponder ways of pursuing these without your partner's knowledge or consent

- you decide that a pregnancy is worth any cost, even if the cost is your health or your marriage

- the thought of stopping treatment is more frightening than the thought of living without children

When desire turns to desperation, as it often does after years of pursuing a pregnancy, it's a good indication that you've lost perspective and need some help. This help may come in the form of professional counseling, spiritual guidance, the support of someone close to you, or stepping back from the infertility treatment experience so that you can regain your emotional and physical health and equilibrium, as well as some objectivity.

After gaining some perspective you may still decide that you need to do one more round of treatment for "closure." But that decision should come from an understanding of what you need to do to be able to move on, rather than from panic and fear. It should come from knowing that you can and will survive even if treatment fails, and from being able to see a possible pregnancy as a bonus, rather than an expectation. After experiencing eight years of fertility investigations and treatments, forty-one-year-old Erin describes it this way:

> We finally got to the point where we realized that we just didn't have control over this and that, as hard as we tried, we couldn't make this happen. It was the realization that if it was meant to be, it would happen and if it wasn't, try as we might, it just wouldn't work. Once we finally got to that point we were able to say, okay, for our own peace of mind we're going to do this one more time and that's it. If it doesn't work so be it—we move on with our lives—and if by some chance it does, then great—it's a bonus.

When You Don't Like the Person You've Become

Another common sign that infertility and the pursuit of a pregnancy may be taking too much of a toll on you and that it's probably time to move on is when you look in the mirror and you realize that you don't recognize the person you see—that you've lost yourself. Or, you may realize that the person you see in the mirror is not someone you particularly like.

Just as infertility can come to encompass a significant portion of your identity, months or years of medical testing and treatments followed by repeated failures can make you feel pretty negative about yourself, your life, and the future. Over time this negativity may start to consume you, and the positive things that used to define you—your energy, your sense of humor, your compassion for others, your sense of efficacy, your commitment to your work and your relationships, your strength, your courage—have been buried under the weight of these repeated losses. You may find that you've let go of many of the things, activities, and relationships that were important to you—many of the things that you valued and that made you feel good about yourself and your life. You may realize that your infertility and feelings of failure have become your constant companions.

This is understandable. For most of us, our self-esteem is connected to our ability to achieve the things that are important to us. However, when producing a child is your goal, and despite all of your best efforts you are unable to make this happen, you are bound to feel pretty lousy about yourself. And unfortunately, without more positive influences to provide some balance, these feelings tend to fester, causing you to feel even more negative and defeated the harder and longer you try to achieve a pregnancy.

So, when you find that each day is defined by the treatment process, and your self-esteem depends solely on your ability to conquer the infertility beast, it's time to step back and assess whether the costs of continuing treatment have become too high. It's time to look in the mirror and see if you recognize the person you see, and if you like the person whose image is reflected there. It's time to assess whether, if you were to achieve a pregnancy, the person in the mirror looks like the kind of parent that you'd want to be.

If you find that you don't like or recognize the person you see, you need to think very seriously about whether it's time to let go—take back your life and, in so doing, take back yourself. Like thirty-six-year-old Nancy describes below, you need to decide what will be left of you, and of the life you've worked hard to create for yourself, if you keep pursuing treatment only to end up with empty arms and an empty life—a life devoid of the things and people who have always been important to you.

> *Every month you're sort of waiting, waiting, and waiting . . .
> only to be disappointed again . . . and before you realize it
> you've put your life on hold for five or six years. Allowing
> myself to really hear the bare facts and discouraging statistics
> was a real turning point. I began to reassess—"What is it I
> really want out of life?" Eventually I had to ask myself how
> much longer I wanted to live my life excluding everything
> that I value about it. How much longer and at what expense
> . . . at the expense of my marriage, my relationship with my
> family, my schooling, my career, my friends . . . how much
> longer and at what cost? I didn't like what I had become. I
> didn't even recognize this desperate person I saw in the
> mirror. So I made a decision. I wrote a letter to the clinic
> saying "No more."*

When You Recognize the Costs to Your Relationship

Another indication that it may be time to consider moving on is when you recognize the tremendous toll that pursuing treatment has taken, and continues to take, on your relationship with your partner. Certainly, working through a crisis like infertility can strengthen your relationship in the long run. Weathering the repeated losses and disappointments, learning to make mutual decisions, and supporting each other as you experience the highs and lows of treatment can definitely increase your confidence in your partner and in your relationship. If you can survive infertility with your relationship intact—and some couples don't—you can probably survive whatever else life throws your way in the future.

These potential gains in your relationship, however, are often offset by a number of significant losses. Many have been discussed throughout this book: communication problems, a loss of sexual pleasure and spontaneity, and serious disagreements about how far each of you is willing to go in your quest to become parents. Other relationship costs include feeling disconnected from your partner; feeling isolated and abandoned, misunderstood, and unsupported; and feeling that your partner is more invested in having a child than she or he is in your relationship.

All of these costs need to be taken into consideration when you're considering whether to continue trying to have a baby. If you find that your communications are now characterized by anger and bitterness, or that there is no longer any laughter, joy, or fun in your interactions with your partner, then perhaps it's time to step back and ask yourself whether the costs of continuing treatment are too high. If you've lost sight of why you wanted to have children with this person to begin with, or you have considered leaving the relationship so that you could pursue a treatment option that your partner is not comfortable with, then perhaps it's time to stop and reconsider your actions. If you look at the current state of your relationship compared to the way it used to be, and you wonder if this is the kind of relationship you'd want to bring children into, then perhaps it's time to decide to move on. After going through four years of fertility treatments, thirty-one-year-old Loretta put it this way:

> One day I was looking at our wedding album and I realized that I didn't recognize the two people in the picture. They were so happy, and we sure weren't. I started to think about how much fun we used to have together, how much laughter

*and promise there was in our lives . . . and that's when I
realized how much we'd lost through all this. That's when I
really became aware of the price we'd paid in trying to have a
child. That's when I came to the realization that it's the
relationship that's important, not the childbearing, not what
society imposes on you—it's the relationship that counts.
That's when I decided it was enough. I wanted to be a parent,
but I wanted to be a parent with my partner—and if we
couldn't have our own child then we'd just have to deal with
that and sort out what we were going to do next—together.*

Interestingly, sometimes it's disagreements over how far each of
you is willing to go in your efforts to become parents, or over how
important parenthood is to each of you, that can keep you stuck pursuing medical treatment solutions. For example, if you are committed
to becoming a parent and are comfortable pursuing other parenting
options such as adoption or third-party reproduction, but your partner is only willing to consider having a child that is biologically
related to both of you, then you may find yourselves locked in the
treatment trap despite the many personal and relationship costs,
because it's your only choice. Or, you may be ready to abandon the
pursuit of treatment, but you agree to continue treatment because of
your partner's wishes and your fear that she or he would leave the
relationship if you stop treatment.

If you find yourselves in situations like these, you probably
need to get some professional help to work through what you both
need and can live with. You may need some help to open up the possibility of other parenting options, or to strengthen your respective
commitments to your relationship, whether or not you become parents together. Or, if through your struggles you've come to realize
that you have very different values and ideas of what you both want
in life and what's important to you, then you should definitely seek
some professional help to sort out whether you've come to a point
where you need to consider going your separate ways.

Confronting Your Fears

Once you realize that you've had enough, the next step in the process
of letting go is facing your fears about an uncertain future. A number
of common fears can keep you from moving forward when you're
trying to decide whether it's time to abandon your efforts to produce
a child. You may be afraid of being overwhelmed by grief and loss

once you stop treatment and have to face the reality of permanent biological childlessness. Certainly the fully weight of this loss is bound to be felt most profoundly when all hope has been extinguished and you give up the fight. However, you've experienced continuous losses throughout this ordeal, from the day you came to realize that you might have difficulty conceiving a child. You've already been grieving the injustice of your infertility, and you have been mourning for the child that you may never have with your partner. So you need not be afraid of hitting an emotional wall. It's a wall you've been up against for a long time now. In deciding to move on, you're actually giving yourself permission to mourn your losses and begin to heal.

Fear of the future can also make it hard to let go and move on. For example, if you're considering adoption, you may be afraid of becoming involved in another difficult, invasive, and time-consuming process—one filled with considerable uncertainty. The thought of having to go through criminal record checks, being assessed by a social worker, being interviewed and selected by a birth mother, negotiating ongoing contact with the birth mother, dealing with the potential genetic or health problems of an adopted child, and of worrying about whether the birth mother will change her mind can seem overwhelming. It can be difficult to consider ending one painful process, only to begin another.

It may be helpful for you to know, however, that although the adoption process has its own challenges and stresses many infertile couples find it to be a much more positive and manageable process—one that, unlike infertility, helps bring them together as a couple in pursuit of a common goal. It also seems to be a process in which many couples feel they have more control over the pace and the outcome. So, if having children is something you're both committed to, and adoption is your next option after fertility treatments, try not to be intimidated by your fears about the trials and uncertainty of another challenging process. The benefits of moving forward may well outweigh the costs, especially if your current medical options have little likelihood of success. Thirty-nine-year-old Richard, an adoptive father, explains it this way:

> You know, it's too bad that we stayed in treatment so long. It
> would have been so much easier, when we found out that
> having babies was not in our life, to just make the decision
> right there and then, "Let's adopt." That would have saved us
> a lot of time and agony—because we'd done enough and we
> just didn't realize it. You get convinced by science that you

need to try everything. But in the long run we decided that being parents is what's important . . . and eventually we realized that the odds of that happening were probably better with adoption. It's just a shame that it took us so long to realize that.

Fear can also keep you from quitting the treatment process if you know that you aren't going to pursue other parenting options like adoption. If you expected to become parents and find you're unable to do so, you may find it difficult to abandon treatment because you're uncertain of what the future will look like if you don't have children. It can be a daunting prospect to have to construct a satisfying future without a road map to guide you. However, many people do construct full lives without kids, and you'll have more personal and relationship resources available to help you with this task, if you don't totally exhaust these in pursuit of a pregnancy. If you are a woman, you may find the book *Never to Be a Mother* by Linda Hunt Anton (1992) to be useful in helping you deal with your feelings of loss and construct a vision of a rich and satisfying life without kids. Couples may find the book *Sweet Grapes: How to Stop Being Infertile and Start Living Again* by Jean and Michael Carter (1989) to be helpful in envisioning a life without children.

What about Regrets?

Another step in the process of letting go and moving on is dealing with concerns about future regrets. Fear of later regrets is another major factor that can keep you locked into the pursuit of treatment. A common question that you've probably asked yourselves several times when deciding on various fertility treatment options is "Will we regret it later if we don't try?" This may not have been an easy question to answer then, and it may not be any easier now. If you previously had any sense that you might someday beat yourself up over the fact that you didn't try a particular treatment option, then even in the face of a poor prognosis you probably went ahead with treatment. Now when you're trying to determine whether to continue treatments, you may again make a decision to go ahead, out of fear of later regrets.

Although you can never be certain about how you're going to feel in the future, part of deciding that it's time, and that it's okay to move on, is deciding that you've done enough. As well as assessing the personal and marital costs of continuing to pursue a pregnancy, be sure to assess whether you feel like you've given it your best shot. If you feel you have, then you probably won't have regrets later. This decision needs to come from an honest assessment of your personal and financial resources and of the potential costs to your relationship. Asking the following questions may be helpful when you are making this assessment:

- Are we confident that we received the best medical advice?

- Within the limits of what we could afford, did we follow the recommendations of the specialists?

- Within the limits of what we could both live with, did we pursue all the available treatment alternatives that had a reasonable chance of success?

- Did we give each treatment option our best effort?

If you can answer yes to these questions, you probably won't have regrets later. Knowing that you've done all you can—that this was indeed a fight well fought—makes it easier to close this chapter of your lives and turn toward the future. As thirty-four-year-old Nathan so accurately points out below, you can't expect yourselves to do more than that.

I feel really good that we tried all that. We really tried everything possible . . . and even though it didn't work, it was worth it . . . because it could have resulted in a baby—it didn't, but it could have. So it's easier to put it to rest knowing we gave it our best shot. We'll always be able to look back without regrets. We did everything we could . . . and you really can't ask more of yourself than that.

Waving the White Flag: Taking Back Your Life

Once you've reconciled yourselves to the fact that you've done all you could to produce a child, be prepared to face a myriad of pretty intense emotions. However you come to the decision that you've done enough and it's time to move on—whether this is something you carefully consider, or whether one day you just wake up and realize that you can't do this anymore—you'll certainly experience a range of mixed emotions.

Relief

Initially, you'll most likely feel relief. Infertility and the pursuit of solutions has taken up a lot of space in your lives, and as hard as it is to face the fact that all your efforts to produce a child were not successful, the thought that you never have to inject yourself with hormones again, give another sperm sample, have a catheter passed through your cervix, have your eggs "harvested," or have anyone slice into your testicles—is an enormous relief. You'll never have to sit in that waiting room looking at all the other desperate faces, and your lives will no longer have to be planned around your next treatment cycle. And, as thirty-seven-year-old Cindy says below, that's a relief.

Thank God that part of our lives is finally over . . . the tests, the appointments, the waiting, the disappointments, the uncertainty. Infertility took up so much space in our lives and now it's finally over . . . and in some ways it's a relief.

Anger

Now that you are no longer focused on being a "good patient" and on doing everything you possibly can to become pregnant, you may be experiencing some pretty intense feelings of anger. You may be angry at the doctors, especially if they were unable to explain what was wrong and why you weren't able to produce a child together. Mark, a forty-seven-year-old attorney, describes it this way:

I went there for answers and didn't get any. I kept saying, "What did we go through this whole thing for if they can't tell us why?" We came out of all this junk, seven years of treatment, still not knowing what was wrong and why it didn't work.

Certainly couples whose infertility remains unexplained tend to have the greatest difficulty letting go. It's very hard to deal with the fact that scientists can put a man on the moon but they can't figure out why you and your partner aren't able to have a child. At least if the doctors had been able to say that there was something wrong with your sperm count, eggs, fallopian tubes, or hormones, then you could chalk it up to fate. But if they simply told you that there is "nothing wrong," it's difficult not to be angry. And the real irony is that, because no one can tell you for certain that you *can't* become pregnant, you may even have to consider using some form of birth

control in the future, when you get to a point in your lives when having children is no longer desirable or safe. So it's understandable that
you might be angry.

Feelings of anger may also surface because this wasn't the way
it was supposed to turn out. After all of the energy and time and
investment you made in trying to have a child together, it can be
hard to deal with the reality that your efforts didn't result in a pregnancy. This is often the point where the injustice of infertility seems
most striking. Thirty-eight-year-old Doreen, a successful business-
woman, put it this way:

> I was angry. There isn't anything else in my life that I've
> worked that hard at really, that I didn't get . . . like I
> deserved to have succeeded. So even though I didn't have the
> energy to do anything else, and I just couldn't do it anymore,
> I was angry. It was like, this isn't the way it is supposed to
> end!

You need to know that these are normal feelings. You've made
a tremendous effort to produce a child, and your investment in the
outcome has been significant. Not being able to produce a child has
already had an impact on virtually all aspects of your life and identity and now it's going to significantly shape the direction your life
takes in the future. The weight of this can feel enormous. Compounding this is the fact that you're probably physically and emotionally exhausted. You've been on an emotional roller coaster for
months or years; when the roller coaster stops, you feel relieved to
get off the ride, but also angry that you're back where you
started—no closer to your goal of having a child, despite your best
efforts.

So give yourself some time to recuperate, physically and emotionally. Pay attention to your health, and get plenty of good nutrition and exercise, even if you feel exhausted or depressed. Avoid the
tendency to begin filling your lives with other activities as a way to
avoid dealing with your feelings. And if your feelings of anger don't
subside on their own as you gain some distance and begin to heal,
then consider what you need to do to work through them so you can
eventually let them go. For example, if you have some residual anger
about how you were treated by some of the medical personnel you
may decide to write a letter to them documenting your feelings and
experiences. You may not ever send the letter, but just putting your
feelings in writing can help you work them through. Or, if your
anger is about the injustice of infertility and directed toward what-

ever higher power you believe in, it may help to talk with your priest or minister about your feelings.

Finally, if your anger seems to be focused at your partner, you need to talk to him or her about you, feelings, or perhaps communicate them in writing. If you find you're not able to resolve these feelings together, then you may need some professional help to work on them. Also, if you're angry at someone else in your life who you feel let you down during your fertility struggles, you need to consider talking to this person about your anger, *if* this relationship is significant enough to you that it's worth salvaging. In so doing, you may find that the relationship ends up being stronger as a result. If not, you've learned something important about whom you can count on when you really need support.

Grief, Hurt, and Loss

The feelings that most frequently underlie anger are hurt, grief, and loss. If you allow yourself to express and accept your anger, you may find that the feelings you really need to work through and express are your feelings of loss over the child you had hoped for and tried so hard to bring into this world. Suggestions for dealing with these feelings are provided in the next section.

A Death in the Family: Mourning Your Losses

Another piece of the emotional work, and a critical step in the process of letting go and moving on, is dealing with the tremendous feelings of loss and grief that being unable to produce a child engender. Although you have been mourning your inability to produce a child for many months or years, and at each period or failed treatment cycle you've cried many tears, there is a finality in choosing to abandon your efforts to produce a child and move on with your life. Similar to the experience of watching a loved one struggle with a terminal illness, although you're prepared for the fact that the person is going to die, you can never fully understand the weight of this reality until it actually happens. As long as the person is alive, there is still hope. As long as you were pursuing solutions to your infertility, there was still hope. But once you have stopped trying to become pregnant—once there is no longer any hope—you need to allow yourself to grieve.

The difficulty with this, however, is that although the child you'd hoped to create, the one who would be the unique expression of the love you share with your partner, was very real to the two of you—she or he existed only in your hearts and minds. Although the loss of this child is very real to you and your partner and is a tragedy in your lives, it is difficult to find concrete ways to acknowledge this loss. After experiencing seven years of fertility treatments, thirty-six-year-old Marilyn found herself asking:

> *Whom do you invite to this funeral where there's no body? There hasn't ever been a body, just a dream. We talked about it and never have been able to come to a resolution as to how we'd mark this passage, the loss of this child that we could or would never have.*

And yet, grieving this loss is a very important part of closing this chapter of your lives and moving forward. Even if you move on to other parenting options, no other child will take the place of the child you've moved heaven and earth to try to create with your partner. And if you do become parents at some point in the future, you need to make space in your minds and hearts for another child. So it is important to deal with this loss. There are many ways that you can mourn the loss of your child.

- Some people find it helpful to write a letter to their child, sharing their unfulfilled hopes and dreams and expectations, and saying good-bye. You and your partner might both do this, and then share your letters with each other. You might consider putting these away in a place that has meaning and significance for you both (perhaps in the family Bible or in the journal you've kept throughout your fertility struggles), so that you can go back and read them at times in the future when you feel a need to reconnect with this part of your lives.

- Rituals can also be very helpful in dealing with your feelings and making your loss more concrete. For example, one couple I worked with, Jim and Leanne, had selected names for the child they had dreamed of creating together—a boy's name and a girl's name. As a way to acknowledge their loss, they bought two helium balloons, wrote the names of their children on these balloons, and, on the beach where they first talked about having children together, they released the two balloons while reading aloud the poem "Burial" by E. Van Clef (Johnson 1984).

- Making your loss more concrete can also be very helpful. For example, after five years of trying to have a baby, Sylvia and Larry were successful getting pregnant through IVF, but their son was stillborn seven months into the pregnancy. The hospital staff took the baby away immediately after delivery and Sylvia and Larry were not given the opportunity to see or name their child. As a way to help deal with their loss, several months later they went back to the hospital and had the medical records changed to reflect the name they had given their son. Then they had a small service at their church and invited their close friends and family members to share with them in a public acknowledgment of their loss.

You need to consider how you and your partner can acknowledge your mutual loss, in a way that is meaningful to you both. Although it can be frightening to confront the depth of your grief, doing so will keep you from getting stuck. It will allow you to come out the other side, healed and whole again. It will allow you to turn toward the future and begin the process of recreating and revisioning your lives together.

"What's Next?": Turning Toward the Future

Finally, once you've had some time to heal physically and emotionally from your experiences—a process that has no particular schedule and may take more time for some people and less for others—you'll find yourselves beginning to consider what the future is going to look like. In essence, you have to rewrite the script of your life. This requires considering your values and reassessing the importance of parenthood in your lives. As Matt, a thirty-seven-year-old carpenter says below, you have to decide what's next and what you need to do to make that happen.

> *In the last five or six years everything else has been put on hold . . . but now the reality is that it's not going to happen—we're not going to be able to become pregnant—so we have to start looking for other ways of enjoying our lives. I've never thought of our lives not including children, but that's what we're faced with and that's what we have to sort out. If it's not going to be kids, what is it going to be? And*

if it still is going to be kids, how are we going to make that happen?

Just as you had to ask yourselves repeatedly over the past several years how badly you wanted to have children together and how far you were willing to go to try to make that happen, you now have to step back and ask yourselves again how important being a parent is in your lives. You need to carefully consider whether you can create a satisfying life and self-image without children being a part of your future. Thirty-three-year-old Kristen, a nursery-school teacher, talks about it this way:

> *For me motherhood has always been a part of my self-concept . . . I always believed that I would be a mum someday. And now that's part of myself that I may have to redefine. And I just don't know whether or not I can. I mean, I've never thought of the other parts of my life or identity being more important than having kids and being a mother. So I need to sort that out.*

You also need to consider whether your relationship can continue to grow if you don't become parents together, and what you need to do to ensure that it does. For example, Maureen and Ron drew confidence from the fact that they were happy and strong as a couple before they experienced infertility, so they knew that they could continue to grow and enjoy their lives as a couple, irrespective of their parental status:

> *We were very happy together as a couple before infertility. Our relationship really worked—that's part of the reason that we decided to try to have kids together. We thought that with such a strong relationship, we'd be good parents. But now that might not happen. And that will be okay, because we're still strong together—we're a unit. Raising kids would have stretched us even further and forced us to grow more, but we're the kind of couple that will always grow anyway because we push ourselves, and that keeps our marriage alive and vital.*

To help accomplish these tasks, you might find it helpful to revisit the exercise in chapter 7 in the section "Infertility as Part, Not All, of Your Identity." Consider the other important roles that define who you are and give meaning to your life, then insert "mother" or "father" into this picture and see how much space that role takes up. If it uses a significant amount of space, perhaps you need to consider other options for making this role a reality, such as adoption or foster parenting, or explore other avenues to include the nurturing of children in your life. If this role takes up only a small amount of space, then perhaps you can consider how you might expand the other roles that give your life satisfaction and meaning.

You may also find it helpful to sit down with your partner and come up with two ten-year plans, one that includes being parents and one that does not. See if you can envision both scenarios and try to fill them out as much as possible, with details such as where you will live and what you will be doing. For example, if you don't become parents will you sell your home and move to a smaller place? Will you stay at your current job or will you consider doing something else? Will you pack it all away for a few years and use this as an opportunity to travel? Will you put more energy into developing other interests and hobbies? Conversely, in your vision of a future that includes being parents, where will you live, what will happen to your careers, and which one of you will take time out from work to stay home with the kids?

Once you've written out the two scenarios, ask yourself which scenario will make you happiest and give you the greatest satisfaction in the long run? Which scenario is most consistent with your values and needs? If you decide together on the scenario that doesn't include being parents, then your work involves redefining your notions of family, envisioning a future that you both can live with and feel good about, and setting some goals to ensure that this future is realized.

If, however, the scenario that works best for you both is the one that includes being parents, then you need to consider how you can make this happen in your lives and begin to take the steps necessary to accomplish this, if you haven't already done so. If adoption is the option you're most comfortable with, you may find the book by Colleen Alexander-Roberts, *The Essential Adoption Handbook* (1993), to be useful. Or, you may wish to contact the organizations listed in Resources. Should you elect to pursue adoption, you also need to find ways to take control of your lives and set some short-term goals that will keep you from feeling stuck or "on hold" again while awaiting the outcome of the adoption process.

You may find that you and your partner don't agree on which scenario fits you best. In talking this through together, explore why each of you is more comfortable with one scenario and less comfortable with the other, and ask yourselves what you fear most about the scenario your partner supports. In these discussions, you may well be able to work through your differences and come to an agreement that meets both your needs. If you can't, however, you may need to seek professional help to sort this through, especially if it seems that you have very different values, or if you find yourselves polarized on this issue with no apparent way to come to an agreement.

Resolution or Reconciliation?

There are a number of books on infertility and adoption, most of which suggest that you need to "resolve" your feelings about your infertility. Many writers suggest that this is necessary to be able to move forward and get on with constructing a satisfying life. Some suggest that it is essential to do this if you are going to be able to accept a child into your hearts and lives who is not genetically related to you. Whether you have terminated your treatment efforts and "adequately resolved" your feelings about your infertility is sometimes used by social workers as a criterion for approval for adoption.

While the notion of resolution is a valid one, I have rarely, if ever, seen anyone who has resolved this issue completely—whether or not they eventually become parents. Even couples who have created families in other ways, and who can say without hesitation that they love their children as much as if they'd given birth to them, don't usually feel that they have completely resolved their feelings about their infertility. Quite the contrary, what they have resolved their feelings about their childlessness; their infertility is still a part of who they are, and it always will be. Forty-year-old Lenore describes it this way:

> I think there will always be that sense that we missed something really important in life. When we listen to other people talk about how awesome the birth of their child was, or when I watch a woman breastfeed her baby, it doesn't level me the way it used to, but sometimes there's this little twinge . . . just a sense of lost opportunity . . . of something very special that we missed.

Whatever path you decide to pursue, it is important to know that your experiences of infertility and your biological childlessness will always be a part of your identities and your lives as well. These experiences have profoundly shaped who you are as a person, and who you are together, as a couple. You may grieve your losses and come to terms with your fate, and, as with mourning the death of someone you loved dearly, in time the pain of the loss will lessen.

However, like an old friend, it will always be a part of your life, and it will surface every now and then to remind you of what you've lost, but also of what you've gained in having survived this very difficult and challenging life experience.

Something Ventured, Something Gained: Assessing Growth and Change

The costs of infertility are many and much has been written about them. Not being able to create a child, experience a pregnancy, or share the birthing experience with your partner is a tremendous loss. And the toll that medical testing and treatment can take on your bodies, lives, and relationship is immense. As you have handled other difficult and challenging life events, however, in time you may also come to see and perhaps even appreciate, some of the strengths you've gained from having lived through and survived infertility.

When you look back at all you've been through, you may be surprised at what you've learned about yourself—about what it really means to be a woman or man. Thirty-eight-year-old Paul, an engineer diagnosed as having no viable sperm, explains it like this:

> *I'm older and wiser. I'm more aware than ever before of a lot of things. Going through infertility has demanded a lot more self-definition than I had previously engaged in. You know there were certain kinds of assumptions that I'd made that were just not true and there was a real process of self-redefinition that I had to go through. If I'd had a good self-image, a good hold on what it meant to be masculine, what it meant to be male, I think infertility would have affected me a lot less—because maleness doesn't come from having kids . . . or having the ability to give a woman a baby . . . it's something else.*

It may surprise you to realize what you've learned about the things you can control in life, and about how to cope with those things that are out of your control. Forty-two-year-old Kimberly put it this way:

> *Both of us have always been very much in control of our lives. All through my life I've had to work very, very hard for whatever I've gotten. So this whole thing with being out of*

control was really hard for me, because no longer was it a situation where if I just worked hard enough I'd get what I wanted—no matter how hard I tried, there still were no guarantees that I'd get a baby. We eventually had to come to terms with the fact that there are things in life we just don't have control over—and that was an important lesson, painful, but important.

When you look back over your experiences you may come to feel that you have grown personally, in your ability to set boundaries and assert yourself and your needs in a way you had not been able to do, before. Pam, a thirty-five-year-old administrator, shares her gains as a consequence of dealing with infertility:

We learned a lot from the medical process and now that I'm much more in a place where I feel I've healed from that, I can let that go. I've learned from that; I can see the pluses, and there have been many. I feel so much more empowered about what I want in my life and how to deal with things when they come up, and that never would have happened if we didn't have this experience . . . I see that as a real positive outcome of something that was very painful.

Through the trials and tribulations of coping with infertility and biological childlessness, you may well have learned some important lessons about relationships, and about who you can count on when the going gets rough. Erica's words reflect these sentiments:

You go through all that grief and aggravation and all the medications, and you give your body over totally to the control of total strangers . . . and when it doesn't work, you feel like you're left with nothing—but that's not true. In fact, you've learned a lot—about yourself, about the medical profession, about faith, about the strength of your relationship, about who you can really count on when the going gets rough.

And finally, if you're like many couples, you will also likely feel that your relationship has been tested, and significantly strengthened, as a result of having to cope with infertility and all that it has come to mean in your lives. Wendy, a thirty-nine-year-old physician, reflects on the benefits to her relationship with her husband Brad:

Going through all this has forced us to become more open about how we feel and to talk about things. It's actually improved our relationship . . . sort of a shared hardship . . .

we're way stronger as a couple now. And we know for sure now that we can count on each other—no matter what!

So, when those feelings of sadness and loss come up, take a moment to acknowledge what you've been through, and then take a moment to think about the way your life, your relationships, your self-image have improved. Reflect on your strength, and courage, and tenacity—in having survived infertility.

Glossary

Amenorrhea. The complete absence of menstruation.

Anovulation. The absence of ovulation.

Antisperm Antibodies. Proteins contained in the man's blood or semen, or in the woman's blood, cervical mucus, or other body fluids that attack the sperm.

Assisted Embryo Hatching. A micromanipulation technique used to assist the embryo to break through the zona (outer shell), thereby facilitating implantation.

Assisted Reproductive Technologies. All fertility procedures that require the laboratory manipulation of sperm, eggs, and/or embryos. (Manipulation and handling are synonymous.)

Azoospermia. The complete absence of sperm in a man's semen.

Basal Body Temperature (BBT). A simple test using a special thermometer to chart the woman's temperature each morning, to assess whether ovulation has occurred.

Blastocyst. The stage of the embryo on the fifth or sixth day following fertilization.

Body Mass Index. A score based on weight and height, used to indicate the risk of illness for most people. A body mass index score from 20 to 25 is associated with the lowest risk of illness.

Chemical Pregnancy. A pregnancy detected through a blood test (increased hCG levels), without the subsequent development of a viable fetus, which is followed by a menstrual period.

Clomiphene Citrate. A nonsteroidal, nonhormonal medication used to induce ovulation in women who are not ovulating but have normal estrogen levels.

Corpus Luteum. The "yellow body" formed in the ovary from an empty follicle that contained the egg before ovulation. Its main function is hormone production.

Cryopreservation. The freezing and storage of embryos during an IVF cycle, for future use or disposition by the couple. The freezing of sperm and possibly eggs.

Donor. A person who provides their eggs, sperm, or embryos to a recipient known or unknown to them, to assist the recipient to achieve a pregnancy.

Donor Egg. Donated eggs of a woman, known or unknown to the recipient, which are transferred to the uterus of the recipient woman after being fertilized with the sperm of her partner.

Donor Embryo. Embryos produced and donated by another couple, to assist an infertile couple to achieve a pregnancy.

Donor Insemination (DI). The use of screened, donated sperm to produce a pregnancy.

Donor Sperm. Sperm donated by a man, known or unknown to the recipient, which are inseminated into the female partner or used with one of the assisted reproductive technologies to fertilize the eggs of the woman.

Ectopic Pregnancy. A pregnancy that implants in a site (usually the fallopian tube) other than the uterus.

Egg Retrieval. Process involving the collection of a woman's eggs using a small needle inserted into the ovarian follicle, following the stimulation of egg production using hormone therapy.

Embryo. The earliest stage in development, after the egg has been fertilized by the sperm and begins the process of cell division.

Endometrial Biopsy. Assessment of the lining of the uterus, based on analysis of tissue scraped from the uterine wall.

Endometriosis. A condition where the endometrial tissue that would normally line the uterus is found growing outside the uterine cavity, potentially impairing fertility.

Endometrium. The lining of the uterus.

Estrogen. Hormones produced by women's ovaries that, among other things, are responsible for the thickening of the uterine lining in preparation for a possible pregnancy.

Follicle-Stimulating Hormone (FSH). A pituitary hormone that stimulates hormone production in both sexes—the growth and release of eggs in women, and the production of sperm in men.

Gamete Intrafallopian Transfer (GIFT). An assisted reproductive procedure that involves the placement of both eggs and sperm into the woman's fallopian tube, prior to fertilization.

Gestational Carrier. A woman who is the recipient of the embryo(s) of another couple, and who carries the fetus through to delivery and relinquishes the baby at birth.

Gonadotropin Therapy. The use of human menopausal gonadotropins (hMG)

Hormone. A chemical substance produced by the body in a specialized gland and transported in the bloodstream to modify the function of other body tissues.

Human Chorionic Gonadotropin (hCG). The hormone produced by the placenta that is assessed to determine if a pregnancy has occurred.

Hysterosalpingogram (HSG). An X-ray of the fallopian tubes and uterus involving the injection of a colorless dye into the opening of the cervix.

Hysteroscopy. A procedure usually conducted under general anesthetic at the same time as a laparoscopy, involving the placement of a small telescope through the cervix to assess the condition of the uterine cavity.

In Vitro Fertilization (IVF). A method of assisted reproduction involving the fertilization of eggs with sperm in a controlled laboratory environment, and the placement of some of the resulting embryos into the woman's uterus.

Intracytoplasmic Sperm Injection (ICSI). A variation of IVF used in cases when a man's sperm is unlikely to fertilize the woman's eggs without being microinjected into the available eggs.

Intrauterine Insemination (IUI). A process whereby the sperm of the male partner is prepared in the laboratory and injected using a catheter into the woman's uterus.

Laparoscopy. A procedure conducted under general anesthetic that requires small incisions in the folds of the skin at the belly button and the pubic hair line for insertion of a scope used for direct visual assessment of the condition of a woman's tubes, ovaries, and uterus.

Luteal Phase. The second half of the menstrual cycle, following ovulation.

Luteinizing Hormone (LH). A pituitary hormone necessary for ovulation and the production of hormones in women, and for the production of testosterone in men.

LH Surge. An increase in the luteinizing hormone released by the pituitary gland to trigger ovulation.

Oocyte. Egg.

Ovulation Induction. Stimulation of ovulation through the use of hormones.

Premature Ovarian Failure. The onset of early menopause triggered by hormone changes.

Progesterone. The hormone secreted by the corpus luteum following ovulation that helps prepared the uterine lining for implantation of a fertilized egg.

Selective Reduction. Also known as multi-fetal pregnancy reduction, this procedure involves the reduction in the number of fetuses a woman is carrying, to decrease the risks of premature delivery and health complications for the remaining fetus(es).

Semen Analysis. Using a high-powered microscope, the man's semen is examined to determine the count (number of sperm), morphology (shape), and motility (movement) of the sperm.

Serum Progesterone Level. A blood test done in the last third of the menstrual cycle to determine ovulation and the development of the uterine lining.

Sperm Count. The number of sperm evident in a man's semen sample using a high-powered microscope.

Sperm Morphology. The shape of a man's sperm detected under a high-powered microscope.

Sperm Motility. The percentage of all moving sperm in a man's semen sample.

Superovulation. Also referred to as ovulation induction, this is the process by which a woman is given ovulation-inducing hormones to facilitate the production and release of multiple eggs.

Surrogate. A woman who is inseminated with the sperm of a man who is not her partner, and who carries the fetus through to delivery and relinquishes the baby to the man and his partner at birth.

Third-Party Reproduction. Any form of treatment that requires the use of the eggs, sperm, embryo, and/or uterus of someone outside of the couple, to achieve and/or carry a pregnancy to term.

Transvaginal Ultrasound. An ultrasound procedure involving the insertion of a vaginal probe to enhance assessment.

Thyroid-stimulating Hormone (TSH) Screening. A blood test used to assess thyroid function.

Unexplained Infertility. The diagnostic description of the status of individuals and couples who are still unable to achieve a viable pregnancy even though the results of all the tests have been normal.

Zona Pellucida. The outer shell of the embryo prior to implantation.

Zygote. An egg in the earliest stage of fertilization, before the cells begin to divide.

Zygote Intrafallopian Transfer (ZIFT). An assisted reproductive procedure that involves the fertilization of a woman's eggs in the laboratory and the immediate transfer of one or more of the resulting zygotes into her fallopian tube(s).

Resources

General Medical Information

Berger, G., and M. Goldstein. 1994. *The Couples' Guide to Fertility*. New York: Doubleday.

Corson, S. L. 1999. *Conquering Infertility: A Guide for Couples*. Vancouver, B.C.: EMIS.

Goldfarb, H., and Z. Graves. 1995. *Overcoming Infertility*. New York: John Wiley & Sons.

Karow, W. G., W. C. Gentry, C. Hsuing, and A. Pope. 1992. *A Baby of Your Own: New Ways to Overcome Infertility*. Dallas: Taylor Publishing Co.

Marrs, R., L. F. Bloch, and K. K. Silverman. 1998. *Dr. Richard Marrs' Fertility Book*. New York: Dell.

Rosenthal, S. M. 1995. *The Fertility Sourcebook*. Los Angeles: Lowell House.

Tan, S.L., H. S. Jacobs, and M. M. Seibel. 1995. *Infertility: Your Questions Answered*. New York: Birch Lane Press.

Medical and Emotional Issues

Cooper, S. L., and E. S. Glazer. *Beyond Infertility: The New Paths to Parenthood*. New York: Lexington Books.

Friedman, R., and B. Gladstein. 1996. *Surviving Pregnancy Loss: A Complete Sourcebook for Women and Their Families.* Boston: Little, Brown and Co.

Harkness, C. 1992. *The Infertility Book: A Comprehensive Medical and Emotional Guide.* San Francisco: Volcano Press.

Johnson, P. I. 1994. *Taking Charge of Infertility.* Indianapolis, Ind.: Perspectives Press.

Mason, M. C. 1993. *Male Infertility—Men Talking.* New York: Routledge.

Mattes, J. 1997. *Single Mothers by Choice: A Guidebook for Single Women Who Are Considering or Have Chosen Motherhood.* New York: Random House.

Nachtigall, R., and E. Mehren. 1991. *Overcoming Infertility: A Practical Strategy for Navigating the Emotional, Medical, and Financial Minefields of Trying to Have a Baby.* New York: Doubleday.

Third-Party Reproduction

Andrews, L. 1990. *Between Strangers: Surrogate Mothers, Expectant Fathers, and Brave New Babies.* New York: Harper & Row.

Clunis, D. M., and G. D. Green. 1995. *The Lesbian Parenting Book.* Seattle, Wash.: Seal Press.

Cohen, C. B., ed. 1996. *New Ways of Making Babies: The Case of Egg Donation.* Bloomington, Ind.: Indiana University Press.

Dutton, G. 1997. *A Matter of Trust: A Guide to Gestational Surrogacy.* Irvine, Calif.: Clouds Publications.

Field, M. A. 1991. *Surrogate Motherhood: Conception in the Heart.* Boulder, Colo.: Westview Press.

Friedeman, J. S. 1996. *Building Your Family Through Egg Donation: What You Will Want to Know about the Emotional Aspects, Bonding, and Disclosure Issues.* Fort Thomas, Ky: Jolance Press.

Ragone, H. 1994. *Surrogate Motherhood: Conceptions in the Heart.* San Francisco: Westview Press.

Seibel, M. M., and S. L. Crockin, eds. 1996. *Family Building Through Egg and Sperm Donation: Medical, Legal, and Ethical Issues.* Boston: Jones and Bartlett.

Vercollone, C., R. Moss, and H. Moss. 1997. *Helping the Stork: The Choices and Challenges of Donor Insemination.* New York: Macmillan.

Adoption

Alexander-Roberts, C. 1993. *The Essential Adoption Handbook*. Dallas: Taylor Publishing Co.

Hicks, R. 1997. *Adopting in America: How to Adopt Within One Year*. Sun City, Calif.: Wordslinger Press.

Johnson, P. I. 1992. *Adopting After Infertility: The Decision, the Commitment, the Experience*. Indianapolis, Ind.: Perspectives Press.

Melina, L. R., and S. Kaplan-Roseqia. 1993. *The Open Adoption Experience*. New York: HarperCollins.

Living without Children

Anton, H. L. 1992. *Never to Be a Mother: A Guide for All Women Who Didn't—or Couldn't—Have Children*. San Francisco: HarperCollins.

Carter, J., and M. Carter. 1989. *Sweet Grapes: How to Stop Being Infertile and Start Living Again*. Indianapolis, Ind.: Perspectives Press.

Flemming, B. 1994. *Motherhood Deferred: A Woman's Journey*. New York: G. P. Putnam's and Sons.

Ireland, M. S. 1993. *Reconceiving Women: Separating Motherhood from Female Identity*. New York: The Guilford Press.

Lisle, L. 1996. *Without Child: Challenging the Stigma of Childlessness*. New York: Ballantine Books.

Hypnosis, Relaxation, and Visualizations

Benson, H. 1975. *The Relaxation Response*. New York: William Morrow & Co.

Benson, H., and E. Stuart. 1992. *The Wellness Book*. New York: Simon & Schuster.

Davis, M., E. Robbins, and M. McKay. 1995. *The Relaxation and Stress Reduction Workbook*. 4th ed. Oakland, Calif.: New Harbinger Publications.

Fanning, P. 1994. *Visualization for Change*. 2nd ed. Oakland, Calif.: New Harbinger Publications.

Hadley, J., and C. Staudacher. 1996. *Hypnosis for Change*. 3rd ed. Oakland, Calif.: New Harbinger Publications.

Kabat-Zinn, J. 1990. *Full Catastrophe Living*. New York: Bantam Dell Books.

Zillbergeld, B., M. G. Edelstein, and D. L. Araoz. 1986. *Hypnosis: Questions and Answers*. New York: Norton.

Zoldbrod A. P. 1990. *Getting Around the Boulder in the Road: Using Imagery to Cope with Fertility Problems*. Lexington, Mass.: The Center for Reproductive Problems.

Books for Friends and Family Members

Johnson, P. I. 1987. *Understanding: A Guide to Impaired Fertility for Family and Friends*. Fort Wayne, Ind.: Perspectives Press.

Clapp, D., and M. Bombardieri. 1994. *How Can I Help? A Handbook for Family and Friends of Couples Going Through Infertility*. Lexington, Mass.: Fertility Counseling Associates.

Organizations Providing Helpful Information

Adoption Council of Canada
P. O. Box 8442, Station T
Ottawa, Ontario, Canada K1G 3H8
(613) 235-1566

Adoptive Families of America, Inc. (AFA)
3333 Highway 100 North
Minneapolis, MN 55422
(612) 537-0316
www.adoptivefam.org

American Society for Reproductive Medicine (ASRM)
1209 Montgomery Highway
Birmingham, AL 35216-2809
(205) 978-5000
www.asrm.com

American Surrogacy Center
638 Church St., N.E.
Marietta, GA 30060
(770) 426-1107
www.surrogacy.com

Childfree Network
7777 Sunrise Boulevard, Suite 1800
Citrus Heights, CA 95610
(916) 773-7178

Infertility Awareness Association of Canada
#523 - 774 Echo Lane
Ottawa, Ontario, Canada K1S 5N8
(613) 730-1322

Infertility Network
160 Pickering Street
Toronto, Ontario, Canada M4E 3J7
(416) 691-3611
www.infertilitynetwork.org

National Adoption Information Clearinghouse (NAIC)
11426 Rockville Pike, Suite 410
Rockville, Maryland 20852
(301) 231-6512

RESOLVE INC.
1310 Broadway
Somerville, MA 02144-1731
(617) 623-0744
www.resolve.org

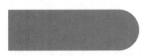

References

Alexander-Roberts, C. 1993. *The Essential Adoption Handbook*. Dallas: Taylor Publishing Co..

American Society for Reproductive Medicine. 2000. *Optimal Evaluation of the Infertile Female*. Birmingham, Alabama: American Society for Reproductive Medicine.

American Society for Reproductive Medicine. 1998. Guidelines for therapeutic donor insemination: Sperm. *Fertility and Sterility* 70:1S-4S.

American Society for Reproductive Medicine. 1998. Guidelines for oocyte donation. *Fertility and Sterility* 70:5S-6S.

American Society for Reproductive Medicine. 1998. Guidelines for embryo donation. *Fertility and Sterility* 70:7S-8S.

Andereck, W. S., D. C. Thomasma, A. Goldworth, and T. Kushner. 1998. The ethics of guaranteeing patient outcomes. *Fertility and Sterility* 70:416-421.

Anton, L. H. 1992. *Never to Be a Mother: A Guide for All Women Who Didn't—Or Couldn't—Have Children*. San Francisco: HarperCollins.

Carter, J. W., and M. Carter. 1989. *Sweet Grapes: How to Stop Being Infertile and Start Living Again*. Indianapolis, Ind.: Perspectives Press.

Cooper, S. L., and E. S. Glazer. 1994. *Beyond Infertility: The New Paths to Parenthood*. New York: Lexington Books.

Corson, S. L. 1999. *Conquering Infertility: A Guide for Couples*. 4th ed. Vancouver, B.C.: EMIS.

Daniluk, J. C. 1996. *Reconstructing a Life: The transition to biological childlessness for infertile couple.* NHRDP# 6610-1959-RH. Ottawa, Ont.: Health Canada.

Domar, A. D. 1997. Stress and infertility in women. In *Infertility: Psychological Issues and Counseling Strategies,* edited by S. R. Leibum. New York: Wiley.

ESHRE Capri Workshop Group. 2000. Multiple gestation pregnancy. *Human Reproduction* 15:1856-1864.

Garcia, J. E. 1998. Profiling assisted reproductive technology: The Society for Assisted Reproductive Technology registry and the rising costs of assisted reproductive technology. *Fertility and Sterility* 69:624-626.

Glazer, E. S. 1990. *The Long-Awaited Stork: A Guide to Parenting After Infertility.* Boston: Lexington Books.

Glazer, E. S., and S. L. Cooper. 1988. *Without Child: Experiencing and Resolving Infertility.* New York: Lexington Books.

Gleicher, N., D. M. Oleske, I. Tur-Kaspa, A. Vidali, and V. Karande. 2000. Reducing the risk of high-order multiple pregnancy after ovarian stimulation with gonadotropins. *New England Journal of Medicine* 343:2-7.

Johnson, P. I. 1984. *An Adopter's Advocate.* Fort Wayne, Tex.: Perspectives Press.

Keye, W. R. 1999. Medical aspects of infertility for the counselor. In *Infertility Counseling: A Comprehensive Handbook for Clinicians,* edited by L. Hammer-Burns and S. N. Covington. New York: Parthenon Publishing Group.

McShane, P. M. Infertility diagnosis and assisted reproductive options: A primer. In *Infertility: Psychological Issues and Counseling Strategies,* edited by S. R. Leibum. New York: John Wiley & Sons.

Seibel, M. M. 1996. Understanding the medical procedures and terminology surrounding reproductive technology. In *Family Building Through Egg and Sperm Donation: Medical, Legal, and Ethical Issues,* edited by M. M. Seibel and S. L. Crockin. Boston: Jones and Bartlett.

————1988. After office hours: In vitro fertilization success rates: A fraction of the truth. *Obstetrics and Gynecology* 72:2.

Society for Assisted Reproductive Technology. 1996. ART registry results: 1994. *Fertility and Sterility* 66:697.

Vercollone, C. F., H. Moss, and R. Moss. 1997. *Helping the Stork: The Choices and Challenges of Donor Insemination.* New York: Macmillan.

World Health Organization. 1992. *WHO Laboratory Manual for the Examination of Human Semen and Sperm-Cervical Mucus Interaction.* Cambridge: Press Syndicate of the University of Cambridge.